Circulation Domination!

Kris McCurry

DEDICATION

This book is dedicated to my daughter. My heart, my soul,
the brightest light I've ever known. My reason for wanting to live
a long and healthy life. I love you, sweetheart.

TABLE OF CONTENTS

TABLE OF CONTENTS CONTINUED

Action

ACKNOWLEDGMENTS

Special thanks to my family and friends for their editing, feedback and never-ending support. Thanks to board-certified physician Dr. Beth Comeau and certified yoga instructor and Feldenkrais Method® practitioner Janice Long of PIOMA Performance Fitness for sharing their knowledge and providing their helpful advice and insight.

CIRCULATION INTRODUCTION

Low energy, fatigue, depression, and chronic illness affect millions. They infiltrate our lives and alter our moods, negatively affecting our relationships, our families, and our jobs—maybe slowly, subtly at first, but progressing a little each year until we feel *old* ... sick, tired, and aged.

Your body's circulatory system is literally your life's blood. Think about your circulatory system feeding your body and mind like water feeds a plant. A plant that gets the proper amount of water flourishes. A plant that gets less water may still live but is less vibrant—it may flower less or produce less fruit. A plant that gets very little water wilts and does not have the energy to produce blooms or fruit. A plant that gets no water wilts and dies.

That's precisely how circulation works in the human body. Your blood carries oxygen and nutrients to every nook and cranny in your body. Healthy, oxygen- and nutrient-rich blood *must* have the ability to reach every cell in your body through healthy blood vessels.

The way we live our lives, our level of physical activity, the foods we eat, and the air we breathe all have a profound effect on our health. Unfortunately, most of us do little things each day that hinder our body's ability to transport healthy blood. Silent and unassuming, these little hindrances will likely go unnoticed for years, or even a lifetime. They may cause many minor health issues for us—fatigue, muscle aches, joint pain, difficulty breathing, colds, the flu, the blues—which we may treat with drugs or simply ignore. When more severe, these hindrances can cause major health issues—chronic fatigue syndrome, chronic bronchitis, heart disease, high blood pressure, depression, and worse yet, heart attack, stroke or even death.

When healthy, oxygen-rich blood faces a roadblock on the way to its intended destination, the body's ability to heal itself is diminished. The greater the roadblock, the bigger the challenge.

When healthy, oxygen-rich blood flows freely, our body performs at its best. Cells, muscles, tissues, and organs get what they need to function in top shape. The body has all the ammunition it needs to fight infection and all the tools it needs to fix what is wrong. We look, feel, and act our best.

With a little knowledge and a little effort, you can make big changes in the way you feel, look, and live.

Circulation Domination! is not rocket science.

Circulation Domination! is not a miracle cure for all of life's ailments.

Circulation Domination! **is** a system for taking control of your body, your health, and your overall well-being. For life.

Circulation Domination! **will** help you heal, thrive, and excel.

CIRCULATION EDUCATION

A quick look at the body's circulatory system, how it works, and why keeping it in tip-top shape is vital to one's overall health and well-being.

To fully understand the amazing impact of circulation on your body and the concepts outlined in this book, let's take a quick refresher on how the circulatory system works. Yes, we learned a lot of this information when we were in school, but do you remember?

Don't worry, this won't have you falling asleep. This is fascinating stuff! And once you fully grasp how crucial GOOD circulation is to your body and how you can improve it NOW, you'll be grateful for the refresher!

OK, so we all know that there are two main elements that keep us alive: circulation (blood flow) and breathing (oxygen). These two work hand in hand to sustain life. Let's take a quick look at how each works.

What is Circulation?

Within the human body, there is a complex system of vessels and muscles that control the flow of blood, or circulation. The primary components of this system are the heart, lungs, arteries, capillaries, and veins.

Circulation begins in the heart when blood leaves the left ventricle and goes into the largest artery in your body—the aorta. The aorta carries oxygen-rich red blood away from the heart through a system of arteries and arterioles (very small arteries). Through these arteries, this oxygen-rich blood, which also contains nutrients from the food we eat, makes its way to every cell in your body. Every cell! Do you know how many cells are in your body? More than 100 trillion!

Arteries, Capillaries & Veins

Blood is carried through the body in blood vessels called arteries, capillaries, and veins.

Arteries *have muscular walls that pump oxygen-filled blood away from your heart to the tissues and organs, like the brain, kidneys, and liver. The further from your heart they are, the smaller they become. At their smallest point, arteries become capillaries.*

Capillaries *are the tiniest blood vessels in our bodies. They connect arteries to veins.*

Veins *bring the "used" blood back to your heart.*

*There are over **60,000 MILES** of blood vessels throughout the human body that feed over 100 TRILLION cells!*

There are literally miles and miles of arteries and arterioles in your body responsible for feeding all of your organs, muscles, tissues, and cells with oxygen- and nutrient-rich blood. Once this healthy blood does its job feeding the body, it makes its way to the ends of the arterioles into your capillaries, where it is ultimately depleted of oxygen and nutrients. This oxygen-poor blood then enters your veins and venules (very small veins)—your venous system—to travel back to the lungs for refueling.

the lungs, carbon dioxide (CO_2) is removed and replaced with the fresh oxygen you inhaled.

So how does air become the oxygen that has such a profound effect in our bloodstream? Let's take a look.

Circulation Oxygenation

Air is taken into your lungs through your nose and mouth. Once in your lungs, the air you breathe dissolves in the water lining of tiny air sacs called alveoli, where it becomes oxygen. Oxygen then clings to red blood cells as they pass through the alveolar capillaries. Oxygen is now in your blood and ready to be taken on a wild ride through your body.

Later in this book, we will look at the lungs and how the simple act of breathing can hinder or help our circulation. (*Hint: most of us are only using a fraction of our lung capacity!*) But for now, let's continue our *Circulation Education*.

To best understand the impact of healthy blood, let's take a quick look at its path through your body.

When blood is pumped away from the heart through the aorta, it enters the carotid arteries and begins its journey to your brain.

Your brain contains *billions* (with a *b*!) of nerve cells responsible for all of the voluntary and involuntary actions in your body.

Thought, behavior, emotion, sensation and movement are all controlled by these nerve cells.

Your brain is made up of several parts – the cerebrum, the cerebellum, the brainstem, and the inner brain. All parts of your brain work together, however each part is responsible for a specific function.

The cerebrum – the largest part of your brain – and all of its parts (the four brain lobes) is responsible for thinking, problem-solving, organization, memory, movement, and sensory information such as taste, touch, smell, and sound.

The cerebellum—located below and behind the cerebrum—is responsible for combining sensory information from your eyes, ears, and muscles to help coordinate movement.

Did You Know...
The brain only represents 2% of one's total body weight, yet it receives 20% of the resting cardiac output that travels through over 400 miles of capillaries!

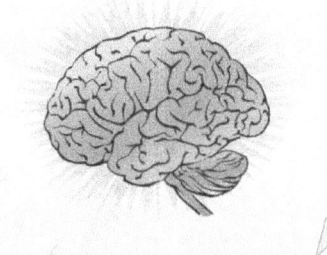

The brain stem—located at the base of the brain—connects the brain to your spinal cord. It controls vital life functions, such as your heart rate, blood pressure, and breathing. It is also important for sleep.

And finally, **the inner brain** controls emotions, memory, and urges like sleeping and eating. The inner brain also regulates body temperature.

Through a complex path of nerves connecting to the rest of your body, these parts of your brain control everything, from your mood to your heart rate.

Wow! With all the amazing things that the brain can do in the blink of an eye (like controlling the blinking of your eyes), you can see why your body sends the best of the best blood there right away!

Later in this book, we will look at the effects—big and small—that diminished blood flow has on the brain.

After it is pumped from your heart, healthy blood makes its way to your brain and upper extremities and travels down to the rest of your body through the descending aorta, behind the heart and down the center of your body. It is sent into the arteries and arterioles to organs, muscles, and every other cell in your body. At the end of its journey, it passes through the capillaries into the venous system on its way back to the heart, and we're back where we started.

Once you understand how your body uses oxygen by way of the bloodstream, you begin to understand how critical maintaining good circulation can be. When it comes to oxygen and blood, if you stop either, you stop life. It stands to reason, then, that if you *hinder* either, you *hinder* life.

The bad news is that NEARLY ALL OF US hinder <u>both</u>, every day. And we don't even know it.

The good news is you won't be too far into this book before you learn some real, easy steps to improving both.

The optimal flow of blood and oxygen is the key to keeping us healthy. Let's take a look at what hindering each can do.

CIRCULATION DETERIORATION

Now that we are all caught up on how circulation works, we can begin to see why keeping it in good shape is so important. So let's take a look at how our circulation can become hindered and cause problems. And if you think your circulation must be healthy just because you eat well and don't smoke, read on.

Although the aging process, a poor diet, and a less-than-healthy lifestyle all play key roles in circulation deterioration, other less obvious factors are often ignored. In this chapter, we will take a look at some of the more obvious culprits, but more importantly, those that are flying dangerously under the radar.

Circulation Vegetation

We're going to start with the one cause of circulation deterioration that most of us are, or have been, guilty of. It's living a sedentary lifestyle, and amazingly, it's the most dangerous. We'll call it *Circulation Vegetation*.

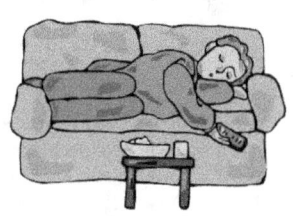

And what we're referring to is not necessarily laziness or CPS (Couch Potato Syndrome!). It can be as quiet and unassuming as what most of us consider a *normal* life—waking up each morning, driving to work, sitting at a desk all day, driving home, fixing a quick dinner, sitting in front of the television for the evening, then heading to bed. Living a sedentary lifestyle simply means not getting enough physical activity, not getting your heart pumping or your body sweating often enough, through walking, running, climbing stairs, or lifting weights.

A study of U.S. adults by the American Cancer Society and published in the *American Journal of Epidemiology* examined the relationship between mortality and leisure time spent sitting versus being physically active. The study showed that people who sat for six or more hours per day were more likely to die sooner than those who sat less.[1]

The study analyzed data from 123,216 adults—53,440 men and 69,776 women—who averaged in their early 60s and were disease-free at the start of the study. During a fourteen-year span, just under 16% of them died (11,307 men and 7,923 women).

The study showed that the more leisure time they spent sitting—watching television, reading, driving, etc.—the more likely they were to have died sooner, particularly from cardiovascular disease, even if they also exercised.

Of those who reported sitting for more than 6 hours a day during their leisure time versus less than 3 hours, women had an approximately 40% higher all-cause death rate, and men had an approximately 20% higher death rate. The combination of both sitting more and being less physically active (more than 6 hours per day sitting and less than 24.5 metabolic

---

[1] Alpa V. Patel, Leslie Bernstein, Anusila Deka, Heather Spencer Feigelson, Peter T. Campbell, Susan M. Gapstur, Graham A. Colditz and Michael J. Thun. "Leisure Time Spent Sitting in Relation to Total Mortality in a Prospective Cohort of US Adults." *American Journal of Epidemiology* 172, no. 4: 419–429, http://aje.oxfordjournals.org/content/172/4/419.full.

equivalent task-hours (METs) of physical activity per week) was associated with a 94% and a 48% increase in all-cause death rates in women and men, respectively, compared with those who reported sitting the least and being the most active (less than 3 hours per day sitting and greater than or equal to 52 MET-hours of physical activity per week).

What To Do

Fixing *Circulation Vegetation* is easy. M-O-V-E. Simply being cognizant of the fact that you need to take any opportunity you can to increase your blood flow is half the battle.

At Work

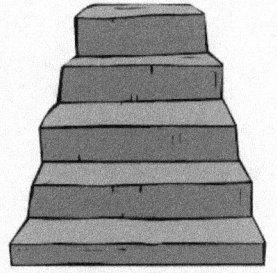

If you work in a building that is several stories high, take the stairs. Even if your office is on the 28th floor, walk up as many flights as you can, and hop on the elevator after that.

Sitting at a computer for long spans of time, as many of us do at work, greatly decreases blood flow. To combat the negative effects of sitting, take frequent, short breaks simply to stand up and move around a bit. Walk to the water cooler or the restroom. Instead of sending an e-mail to your coworker in the next office, take a walk and have a real, face-to-face conversation! There are even simple exercises that you can do at your desk while not breaking your work stride (see The Fitness Flex in Chapter 8).

Talk to your employer about offering free or supplemented gym memberships or fitness classes, such as yoga, during work hours. A 45-minute yoga break a few times a week will not only do wonders for the health and mindset of the staff, but it will likely increase their overall productivity as well!

At Home

When you first get up in the morning, take a few minutes to care for your circulation. Drink a glass of water, do some deep breathing and give your body a good stretch. If you're feeling really energetic and have the time, take a brisk walk, or pop in an exercise video and get that blood moving!

If you have kids at home or nearby, play! No matter how old you are, playing games with young children is sure to get your blood moving.

In the evening, take some time to walk around your neighborhood. If that is not an option, take some time to walk up and down steps or around your yard a few times. If you are feeling really motivated, do a DVD fitness video.

Being physical not only helps your circulation, it can help you get a good night's rest also.

Circulation Asphyxiation

In Chapter 1, we learned how healthy, oxygenated blood is transported throughout the body and how this healthy blood plays a vital role in normal body function.

Normal, healthy blood-oxygen levels are between 95% and 100%. Adult smokers who are otherwise "healthy" could have levels as low as 90%. People who suffer from COPD (Chronic Obstructive Pulmonary Disease) may have levels as low as 85%.

Without the proper amount of oxygen in your bloodstream, your body's cells—and thus your tissues, muscles, and organs—are being asphyxiated. Because blood oxygenation happens in the lungs, it's important to look at the different types of lung conditions that hinder blood oxygenation.

COPD, which includes asthma, chronic bronchitis, and pulmonary emphysema, has been diagnosed in an estimated 16 million Americans, with an additional 16 million who may be undiagnosed.[2] Additionally, others suffer from different types of lung disorders, including cystic fibrosis, interstitial lung disease, pneumonia, pulmonary hypertension, pulmonary embolism, pulmonary sarcoidosis, tuberculosis, and lung cancer.

Not only is this information scary, it's costly. COPD alone costs the U.S. economy an estimated $31.9 billion each year.[3] That's quite a list, and quite a lot of people suffering from low blood-oxygen issues.

Smoking

When most of us think of the disease that will most likely take the life of a smoker, we think of lung cancer. It is interesting to note, then, that smoking can also cause coronary heart disease, stroke, abdominal aortic aneurysm, acute myeloid leukemia, cataracts, pneumonia, periodontitis, and bladder, esophageal, laryngeal, oral, throat, cervical, kidney, stomach, and pancreatic cancers.[4]

Cigarettes contain 4,800 chemicals (69 of which are known to cause cancer); however, two chemicals in particular are to blame for their profound effect on blood vessels—nicotine and carbon monoxide. Nicotine is a stimulant that raises the heart rate. As you smoke, arteries throughout the body constrict, elevating blood pressure and making it more difficult for the heart to pump blood through the vessels. This increased heart rate is part of the addiction of smoking—it provides a

---

[2] Petty, T. L. "A new national strategy for COPD." *Journal of Respiratory Diseases* 18, no. 4 (1997): 365–369.

[3] American Lung Association Fact Sheet: Chronic Obstructive Pulmonary Disease (COPD), Sept. 2000. New, unpublished data from the National Heart, Lung and Blood Institute offers an estimate of $30.4 billion.

[4] American Lung Association General Smoking Facts, http://www.lungusa.org/stop-smoking/about-smoking/facts-figures/general-smoking-facts.html.

quick rush, tricking the smoker into thinking he needs a smoke as a pick-me-up.

In order to combat these nasty side effects, the heart must work harder. To work harder, the heart needs additional oxygen, which it must receive from oxygenated blood. But wait—there was carbon monoxide in that cigarette. Carbon monoxide competes with oxygen for hemoglobin, making it difficult for the hemoglobin to deliver healthy blood to our body tissue. The heart is faced once again with working even harder to get the right amount of oxygenated blood to the tissue.

This vicious cycle is the cause of decreased circulation, which in turn is the cause of a vast number of ailments and diseases.

What To Do

If you suffer from *Circulation Asphyxiation*, there are several things you can do to breathe easier and increase the oxygen in your bloodstream.

If You Smoke

Stop. Easier said than done, I know, but it's an absolute must for good health. If you can't do it on your own, see your doctor for a prescription that can help, or join a support group or forum.

Increasing Lung Capacity

Another way to breathe easier is to incorporate breathing exercises into your daily routine. Most of us are shallow breathers. We use only the upper 20% or so of our lungs. And if you're an ex-smoker, have asthma, or feel as though breathing is often difficult, that upper 20% isn't enough to keep the right amount of oxygen flowing into your bloodstream.

The good news is, you can increase your lung capacity with some simple lung exercises.

Lung Exercise #1 – The Relaxer

Lie on a flat surface with your head slightly elevated (a pillow works well). Breathe in through your nose, allowing your stomach to expand to take in as much air as you can. Once you think you have taken in all you can, force in some more! Get as much air into your expanded lungs as possible, and hold it there as long as you can.

When exhaling, do so through pursed lips (as if you're blowing out a candle).

Take several normal breaths, then repeat the deep breathing 4 more times. All in all, this should only take you a few minutes, and it is a great exercise to do before you get out of bed in the morning and when you lie down at night.

Lung Exercise #2 – The Power Breather

Stand with your feet hip-width apart and your hands at your sides. Breathe in through your nose and fill your lungs with as much air as possible. Allow your stomach to expand to give your diaphragm and lungs as large an area as needed. Once your lungs feel full, breathe in some more until you can't take in any more air. Hold the air in as long as possible. When you can no longer hold it in, 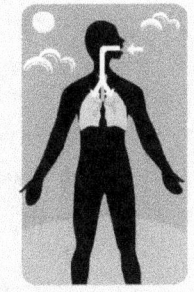 force the air out quickly through your mouth. Keep exhaling and cough to force all of the air out completely.

Once the air is forced out, keep it out for as long as you can. When you can no longer keep it out, bring air back in quickly through an open mouth, as if gasping. Breathe normally for several breaths. Repeat the Power Breather 4 more times.

If at any time you begin to feel dizzy, stop. Resume only when feeling normal, and decrease the intensity of the exercise until your lungs have had a chance to build up strength.

Go Cardio

Cardiorespiratory exercise is a great way to get your lungs in tip-top shape. Power walking, jogging, running, swimming, fitness classes, and even dancing are perfect for getting blood pumping and your lungs working. To stay healthy, adults need at least 150 minutes per week of moderate-intensity cardio activity, and a combination of muscle-strengthening activities at least twice each week. See Physical Activity in Chapter 8 for more helpful information on cardio exercise.

Circulation Intoxication

If you consume alcohol on a regular basis, there is good news and bad news when it comes to circulation.

The **good news** is that consuming small amounts of alcohol of any type—not just red wine—relaxes blood vessels, reducing the amount of work the heart must do.

The **bad news** is that the good news is limited to small amounts of alcohol. If you enjoy consuming more than one drink, the benefits turn from positive to negative.

Researchers at the Peter Munk Cardiac Centre of Toronto General Hospital conducted a study that showed that after one drink, blood vessels became more relaxed. But after two drinks, the heart rate, the amount of blood pumped from the heart, and the action of the sympathetic nervous system all increased. Simultaneously, the ability of the blood vessels to expand in response to the increase in blood flow was diminished, decreasing circulation[5].

---

[5] American Heart Association. "Light to moderate drinking linked to fewer heart problems in male bypass patients, study finds." *ScienceDaily* (November 15, 2010), http://www.sciencedaily.com/releases/2010/11/101114161823.htm (accessed September 18, 2011).

Circulation and Medication

Increased or decreased circulation can be side effects of medication. However, there are simply too many drugs on the market to list those that cite increased or decreased blood flow as a side effect.

If you suffer from high blood pressure, have other circulatory or heart-related health issues, or suffer from Erectile Dysfunction (ED), you may already be on medication that is designed to regulate or increase blood flow. The good news is that the steps outlined in this book will aid in the effectiveness of these circulation-stimulating drugs (see Circulation Sensation in Chapter 3).

What To Do

If you take medication of any kind – prescription or over-the-counter – read the drug information and possible side effects. If a decrease in blood flow is a side effect, talk to your doctor about how this may be affecting your current and long-term health.

Additionally, if you are on any medications, before implementing any major changes in your diet or exercise routine, speak to your doctor and discuss your plans and goals.

Who knows, maybe the steps you take to improve your cardiovascular health will lessen or even eliminate your need for medication altogether.

CIRCULATION CAUSATION

A look at how circulation – good and bad – affects the mind and body.

Circulation and Depression

Oxygen is essential for brain function: 20% of the body's oxygen is used by the brain, yet the brain represents only about 2% of the average body's weight. Your arteries (carotid and basilar) are responsible for transporting oxygen-rich blood from your heart to your brain. A lack of blood flow to any part of the brain can result in pain, depression, or even a stroke.

Along with other factors, such as chemical imbalance, studies show that decreased blood flow to the lower brain can cause depression. Antidepressant medications, in addition to targeting certain neurotransmitters, help to increase blood flow to the lower brain.

As we age, our circulation naturally lessens. We move a bit slower and therefore aren't requiring as much blood flow. Veins and arteries become less flexible. Plaque and cholesterol buildup can occur, causing blood flow to slow or even become blocked.

Coincidentally (or not), the National Institute of Mental Health reports:

- Older Americans are disproportionately likely to die by suicide. Although they comprise only 12% of the U.S. population, people age 65 and older accounted for 16% of suicide deaths in 2004.

- 14.3 of every 100,000 people age 65 and older died by suicide in 2004. In the general population, the rate was about 11 per 100,000.

- Non-Hispanic white men age 85 and older were most likely to die by suicide. They had a rate of 49.8 suicide deaths per 100,000 persons in that age group.[1]

Supporting this theory even further, a study by the American Heart Association found that depression is commonly present in patients with coronary heart disease (CHD) and is independently associated with increased cardiovascular morbidity and mortality. *Depression and Coronary Heart Disease*[2] reviews the evidence linking depression with CHD and provides recommendations for healthcare providers for the assessment, referral, and treatment of depression.

---

[1] National Institute of Mental Health, Suicide in the U.S.: Statistics and Prevention, NIH Publication No. 06-4594 http://www.nimh.nih.gov/health/publications/suicide-in-the-us-statistics-and-prevention/index.shtml#adults.

[2] "Depression and Coronary Heart Disease", *Circulation* 2008, 118:1768-1775: September 29, 2008, Judith H. Lichtman, J. Thomas Bigger, Jr, James A. Blumenthal, Nancy Frasure-Smith, Peter G. Kaufmann, François Lespérance, Daniel B. Mark, David S.Sheps, C. Barr Taylor and Erika Sivarajan Froelicher http://circ.ahajournals.org/content/118/17/1768.full.pdf

What To Do

The Center for Disease Control and Prevention (CDCP) estimates that as many as 1 in 10 adults in the U.S. report suffering from depression. And those are just the people who report it. The statistics may actually be much higher. If you are or believe you are suffering from depression, first and foremost, see your doctor and develop a plan for caring for your depression.

Once that is done, help increase your success rate even more by making sure the circulation to your brain is in tip-top shape.

3 Quick Tips for Increasing Blood Flow to the Brain

1. Breathe! Taking deep breaths increases oxygen in the blood, providing more to feed your brain. Cardio-focused exercise, such as walking, running, and swimming, also increases the amount of oxygen in your blood. Want to do well on that big test or in that important meeting? Increase blood flow to your brain with several minutes of walking up and down a flight of stairs first!

2. Take Vinpocetine, sold under the brand names Cavinton and Intelectol. It increases blood flow to the brain and is used in Europe to treat cerebrovascular disorders. Vinpocetine is derived from the periwinkle plant, and research shows that it is a powerful memory enhancer.[*]

3. Incorporate gingko biloba into your diet. The leaves of the gingko biloba tree have been proven to increase blood flow to the brain and are widely marketed as a memory enhancer. Inexpensive and readily available, gingko biloba comes in capsules and as a tea.[*]

* Before taking any supplements, be sure to check with your doctor, especially if you are currently on any prescription medication.

Circulation Aggravation

We all get aggravated, angry, or stressed from time to time. It's a normal human response to certain situations. Anger, however, can be harmful to your circulation. During periods of anger, your body releases the hormone adrenaline into the bloodstream and your blood pressure rises temporarily. Prolonged periods of anger that cause an increase in heart rate and blood pressure damage artery walls, and may be a contributing factor to heart disease.

Did You Know ...
Your body releases adrenaline when you are angry to prepare you to deal with the situation. It's telling you to either confront it or run away, and is known as your "fight or flight" response.

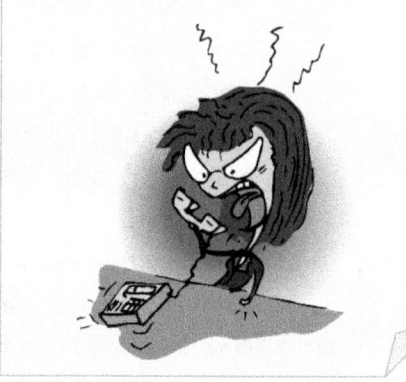

When we think about the times we are the least aggravated, and the happiest, it's usually when we are physically feeling our best. Think about it. When your body feels good—you're alert, well-rested, energized, no aches or pains—your mood is also good.

Things like fatigue, low energy, headaches, muscle pain, or cold hands and feet make us feel *off*. And when we feel off, we tend to sweat the small stuff. I mean, how cranky are we when we're tired? We snap at our kids, our coworkers, our significant others. We get angry at what may seem like the smallest thing.

So, what if we feel bad most of the time? What if we're walking around all day, every day just one bad driver away from a complete meltdown? Not a great way to live.

What To Do

Feelings of aggravation may come on strong (and often!), but they don't have to control you. Recognizing that you're getting angry or aggravated is the first step. I honestly believe that some people spend so much of their life in a constant state of aggravation that they don't even realize it!

If you've recognized that your "blood is starting to boil," try these tips for controlling anger from the American Psychological Association[3].

- Breathe deeply, from your diaphragm; breathing from your chest won't relax you. Picture your breath coming up from your "gut."

- Slowly repeat a calming word or phrase like "relax" or "take it easy." Repeat it to yourself while breathing deeply.

- Use imagery; visualize a relaxing experience, from either your memory or your imagination.

- Non-strenuous, slow, yoga-like exercises can relax your muscles and make you feel much calmer.

- Practice these techniques daily. Learn to use them automatically when you're in a tense situation.

---

[3] American Psychological Association, "Controlling Anger Before it Controls You," http://www.apa.org/topics/anger/control.aspx.

Circulation Exhaustion

The muscles in your body are responsible for all of your body's movement—voluntary and involuntary. Your heart is a muscle. Muscles control your breathing, blinking, swallowing, walking, talking, laughing, and every little movement in between.

Blood flows to your muscles through small arteries and arterioles. Each muscle fiber is surrounded by several capillaries. In order for your muscles to function properly, they require healthy, oxygenated blood. Therefore, it stands to reason that when circulation is poor, healthy blood is not fully reaching and replenishing those muscles.

When muscles are not fed with healthy blood, they become tired and weak. Now picture ALL of your muscles being adversely affected by poor blood flow. No wonder we feel tired!

What To Do

Quick Tips on Increasing Blood Flow to Muscles

The first step to increase blood flow to your muscles is to simply *move*! Sitting or lying around as a way of life is a vicious cycle. You lie around because you're tired, but you're tired because you're lying around!

Make a conscious effort to add movement to your day. Walk, run, dance, play—whatever it is, just do something to get that blood going!

Another quick and easy step in helping to increase blood flow to your muscles is drinking water. The consumption of healthy amounts of water has many benefits, including providing much-needed oxygen to your blood, thus increasing blood flow. Plus, the more water you drink, the more you'll have to get up, get moving, and go to the restroom!

Circulation and Hospitalization

By now you see how circulation affects every part of your body. The deprivation of blood flow, whether sudden or over time, can have both subtle and catastrophic consequences.

And while fatigue and depression may not put you in the hospital, a stroke or heart attack surely will.

Heart Disease

The Center for Disease Control lists heart disease is the #1 cause of death in the nation, and estimates that one American each minute will die from a coronary event[4]. In hospitals, millions of patients are treated each year for a wide range of heart-related issues, including hypotension (low blood pressure), hypertension (high blood pressure), cardiac obstruction, and cardiac arrest.

While we may think that heart disease is predominantly a male issue, according to the American Heart Association, "more women die from heart disease, stroke and other cardiovascular disease (CVD) than men, yet many women do not realize they are at risk. These diseases kill more women each year than the next five causes of death combined."

Stroke

A stroke is a disruption in the flow of blood through the brain, which damages brain tissue. There are two types of stroke. The most common type—ischemic stroke—results from blockage of an artery. Sometimes called a mini-stroke, a transient ischemic attack (TIA) temporarily disrupts blood flow through your brain. The other type—hemorrhagic stroke—occurs when a blood vessel leaks or bursts.

---

[4] National Center for Chronic Disease Prevention and Health Promotion, Division for Heart Disease and Stroke Prevention, http://www.cdc.gov/features/heartmonth.

What To Do

To be sure that you are not at risk for a heart attack or stroke, the best thing to do is see your doctor regularly, particularly if you have a family history of high blood pressure, heart disease, high cholesterol, or stroke. Get regular physicals, and share any concerns you may have with your doctor.

The Truth About Aspirin

Often times, an aspirin a day is recommended to help lessen the likelihood of a heart attack. Daily use of aspirin can have serious side effects, including internal bleeding, and is not right for everyone. According to the Mayo Clinic, aspirin is recommended only if you've had a heart attack or stroke, or you have a high risk of either.

Eat Right and Exercise

The best medicine for warding off a heart attack or stroke is a healthy lifestyle. Eating right, exercising, and being in tune with how your body works is the key to a long and healthy life.

Circulation and Amputation

Harsh, yes! But it's a reality. Ask any physician and s/he will tell you that the majority of patients who lose limbs to amputation have done so because the circulation in those limbs was gone. No blood flow, no life.

The diminishing of arterial circulation—otherwise known as atherosclerosis—is the #1 reason for amputation. Atherosclerosis prohibits the proper flow of oxygenated blood to your life-sustaining organs and other parts of your body. Atherosclerosis, which often has no warning signs, can result in different diseases, including carotid artery disease (stroke), peripheral vascular disease (peripheral numbness and pain), and coronary artery disease (heart disease, angina, dyspnea, arrhythmia, and heart attack).

Circulation Beautification

The skin is the largest organ in the human body. Its health and well-being are affected by many exterior factors, such as sun exposure and hygiene. But the two most important factors in ensuring that your skin is healthy are circulation and hydration.

Blood is carried to the skin through millions of capillaries. All you have to do is get a little paper cut to realize that there is blood flow all the way up through the many layers of the epidermis. Therefore, does it not make sense that when your circulation is diminished, your skin, hair, and nails suffer? Of course!

Peruse the many beauty treatments on the market today, and you will see several that increase circulation to the skin's surface. That's because by bringing the blood to the surface, you are bringing with it oxygen and nutrients essential to healthy skin.

Water is another major beauty aid. Water not only helps to cleanse the body of toxins and aid in digestion, but also helps to circulate your blood for healthy blood flow to the skin.

For more on how circulation affects the skin, Dr. Beth Comeau, a board-certified physician and medical aesthetic practitioner practicing in Maryland, offers insight and advice. Dr. Comeau provides a variety of treatments, including laser treatments, aimed at increasing blood flow to the outermost portions of the skin.

Dr. Beth Comeau Offers Helpful Skin Advice

"Blood flow to the skin is so important. It affects how our skin looks on the surface and how it acts beneath the surface.

"One of the clear indicators of how blood flow to the skin affects how our skin looks is smoking. When I see patients who smoke, they tend to have skin that is not as vibrant as those who do not. Smoking constricts the blood vessels that deliver blood flow to the skin and thus inhibits nutrients and antioxidants from reaching the skin's surface.

"When we deplete our fibroblasts (the cells in the skin that produce collagen) from receiving oxygen and vital nutrients, healing is diminished and your fibroblasts cannot make new collagen as quickly. This results in skin that is dull and lacking in elasticity.

"When it comes to skin having a youthful, vibrant appearance, exercise and stimulating blood flow to the skin is a tonic for antiaging! Good blood flow helps remove toxins and provides hydration and nutrients to the skin, increasing its vitality.

"To make sure your skin is being fed properly from now on, take care of your circulation! If damage has already been done, never fear. Advancements in medical aesthetics, as well as making lifestyle changes, can help increase circulation and bring back a more youthful you."

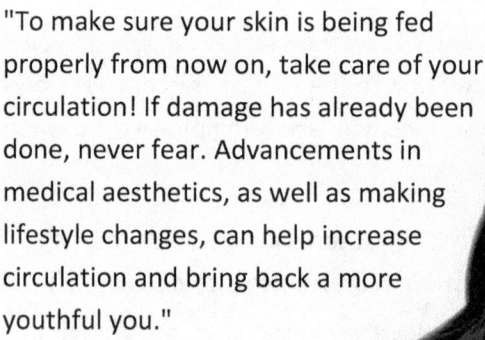

Beth Comeau, MD
www.BethComeauMD.com

What to Do

Although skin type is hereditary, there are things you can do to improve the quality of your skin, no matter what skin type you have.

5 Tips to Great Skin

1. Start by keeping your skin well hydrated. Drink plenty of water, and follow a skin-care regimen that nourishes your skin.

2. Use sunscreen daily—even during the winter! The sun's ultraviolet rays create free radicals that damage the skin and cause premature aging and skin cancer. Use a daily moisturizer that includes sunscreen on any part of your skin that will be exposed to sunlight.

3. Brush your skin while bathing. In the shower or bath, use a natural horse-hair brush and stroke wet skin with short strokes toward your heart. Start at your feet and work up to your chest. The bristles help stimulate blood flow to the surface of the skin, and help to exfoliate dead skin.

4. Get a massage. Massaging skin helps bring circulation to the surface and helps release toxin buildup. It also happens to be a wonderful mood-enhancer!

5. Visit your doctor for regular skin checkups. Be sure to have any suspicious moles or lesions checked annually. Also, regularly check your skin on your own, and see your doctor if you find anything suspect.

6. To help reverse the look and depth of wrinkles, and to treat aging skin, consult a medical aesthetic practitioner. Advancements in laser skin treatments can help restore lost circulation and boost natural collagen production.

Circulation Sensation

Sensation. Touch. Feel. Pleasure. Your fingertips, hands, feet, toes, lips, and yes, the sexually stimulated areas of your body are greatly affected by blood flow.

Sexual arousal depends on an increase in blood flow. That is why fatigue can play such a large factor in arousal. Foreplay, in fact, is all about circulation. A touch in the right place, closeness, a kiss, are ways of getting your heart beating faster and your blood moving in the right direction.

An erection is not possible without an increase in blood flow to the penis. If you and your partner have tried any of the erectile dysfunction (ED) products on the market today, you are well aware of this phenomenon already! ED medications do their job by increasing blood flow. Patients not only become aroused, their skin will also become warm and flush through the increase in circulation.

In fact, recent research from the Mayo Clinic shows that the symptoms of ED can be reduced by improving one's lifestyle. Lowering your cholesterol, controlling blood pressure, losing weight, and exercising increases circulation and thus reduces the symptoms of ED.

Although men are more likely to seek treatment for the symptoms of ED than the symptoms of potential heart disease, a report in the *Archives of Internal Medicine* revealed some statistics that may have them making heart-healthy changes. It stated that men with ED who either made lifestyle changes to lower their risk of heart disease or took medications to control their high cholesterol or blood pressure were 2.5 times more likely to see improvements in their sexual function over a period of at least six weeks than those who didn't make the heart-healthy changes.

The study also showed that men who took ED medication and took steps to improve their lifestyle reported even more benefits to sexual function[5]. What's more, urologists at the Mayo Clinic are starting to refer younger patients with ED to heart specialists to check for underlying heart disease.

It makes perfect sense, doesn't it? Our arteries are all connected. Improve the blood flow, and improve *everything*.

Orgasms in both males and females are also greatly enhanced by healthy blood flow. So, if looking good and feeling good weren't enough of a reason for *Circulation Domination!*, this should be!

What to Do

According to Harvard Medical School, ED has many culprits, including:

- Vascular disease
- Neurological problems
- Psychological factors
- Metabolic syndrome
- Diabetes
- Prostate cancer
- Benign prostatic hyperplasia

- Medications
- Hormonal disorders
- Weight
- Exercise
- Smoking
- Alcohol or substance abuse[6]

If you or your partner suffer from ED, the first thing to do is speak to your physician. In some cases, ED can be a barometer for other health issues. Therefore, treating it may just save your life—not to mention give you back one of life's greatest pleasures.

---

[5] Alice Parks, "To Help Erectile Dysfunction, Treat the Heart," *Time*, http://healthland.time.com/2011/09/13/to-help-erectile-dysfunction-focus-on-the-heart/.

[6] *What to do about Erectile Dysfunction*, prepared by the editors of the Harvard Health Publications in consultation with Michael Philip O'Leary, MD, Senior Surgeon at Brigham and Women's Hospital and Professor of Surgery at Harvard Medical School, 38 pages (2009).

CIRCULATION ATTENTION

Poor circulatory health puts you at risk for heart disease, stroke, depression, and so much more. By assessing your Risk Factor, you can help determine how aggressive you want to be in achieving Circulation Domination!

Now we know how circulation may have a hand in those annoying little ailments, or worse yet, those larger health issues. Just for fun, let's see what our level of risk may be for poor circulation. Let's take the **Risk Factor** quiz.

Read the questions on the following page and circle the Risk Factor numbers that match your answers. Enter your scores for each question in the Your Score column. Add your numbers up at the end and enter the total in the Total Score column. Then compare your Risk Factor number to the Risk Factor Scores on the following page.

Note that some Risk Factor numbers for Question 6 are <u>negative</u> numbers, meaning that you can actually *improve* your score by subtracting these numbers if you have incorporated moderate to intense cardio exercise into your weekly routine!

What's Your Risk Factor?

1.	What is your age?	18-25	26-35	36-45	46-55	56-65	66-75	75+	YOUR SCORE
	Risk Factor #	1	2	3	4	5	6	7	
2.	Describe your weight.	Under Weight	Healthy Weight	Over Weight	Obese				
	Risk Factor #	2	1	3	7				
3.	How much do you smoke?	Never	Quit 5+ years ago	Quit in the last 5 years	Smoke Some	Smoke Moderately	Smoke Heavily		
	Risk Factor #	1	2	3	5	6	7		
4.	How much alcohol do you drink?	None	Less than 1 drink per day	1–2 drinks per day	2–3 drinks per day	More than 3 drinks per day			
	Risk Factor #	1	1	2	5	7			
5.	How much do you walk each day*?	Never	Less than 1 mile	1–3 miles	3–5 miles	More than 5 miles			
	Risk Factor #	7	5	3	2	1			
6.	Frequency of moderate to intense cardio exercise	Never	1 day per week	2–3 days per week	4–5 days per week	5+ days per week			
	Risk Factor #	4	2	-2	-4	-6			
7.	Describe your overall diet**	Extremely healthy	Healthy	Somewhat healthy	Not healthy	Very unhealthy			
	Risk Factor #	1	2	3	5	7			
	Total Score								

*To help determine how much you walk each day, see "Walking" on page 34.
**To help determine how healthy your diet is, see "What is a healthy diet?" on page 34.

Risk Factor Scores

Below you will find score ranges to help calculate your Risk Factor. The lower your score, the more likely you are to have good circulation. If your score is high, don't be discouraged. Follow the tips in this book to make positive changes to help you achieve *Circulation Domination!* Then, come back and take this quiz again to see how you've improved.

This quiz is just for fun and is not meant to make a diagnosis or take the place of any medical examination. Prescription medications and environmental factors may have an additional impact on your circulation. No matter what your score—good or bad—you are encouraged to speak to your doctor about your current health and how to make improvements for optimum circulation.

Risk Factor Scores

8–15 You're in *Circulation Domination!* Keep up the good work!

16–25 You might be feeling occasionally sluggish or down. Your circulation may need just a little work. But with some small changes, you should be in top shape in no time!

26–40 You are probably feeling fatigued, maybe a little depressed, or you might be suffering from circulation-related health issues. Follow the simple tips in this book and talk to your doctor about lifestyle changes that can help you gain better control of your health.

41+ You may be at high risk for circulatory health issues, such as high blood pressure, heart disease, or stroke. It's a good idea to see your doctor and work on ways to improve your overall health.

*Walking

When it comes to the amount of walking you do per day, you might be surprised. The average person's stride length is about 2.5 feet, meaning that within about 2,000 steps, you have walked a mile. Even someone living a sedentary lifestyle can average 1,000–3,000 steps per day, so chances are you're walking at least a few miles per day. To find out for sure, purchase a pedometer and wear it for a week, then average out your distance.

**What is a healthy diet?

Extremely Healthy: All whole grains, organic fruits and vegetables, no trans fats, no refined sugar or white carbs, organic low-fat meats (fish, chicken, pork), no processed foods, low sodium.

Healthy: All whole grains, fruits, vegetables, no trans fat, no refined sugar or white carbs, low fat meats, limited processed food, low sodium.

Somewhat Healthy: Mostly whole grains (occasional white carbs), fruits, vegetables, limited refined sugar, limited processed food, limited red/processed meat, limited sodium intake.

Not Healthy: No whole grains, refined sugar and white carbs, limited fruits and vegetables, processed foods, some trans fats, any meats, no attention to sodium intake.

Very Poor: A steady diet of refined sugar, white carbs, fried foods, fatty meats, processed foods, trans fats, no attention to sodium intake.

How did you score?

If you scored well, congratulations! You're already taking the right steps to live a long, healthy life. If you didn't score well, don't be discouraged. The only item on the Risk Factor quiz that can't be changed is your age!

CIRCULATION NUTRITION

We all know the old saying, "You are what you eat." But the reality is that most of us don't know exactly *what* we eat. We often think we're eating healthy, but a number of items hidden in food can fly under the radar and become a danger to our health.

Our society is structured for busy lifestyles. Over the past seventy-plus years, food companies have gone to great lengths to make eating easy. The process of making foods quick and easy to prepare has resulted in food that is, well, processed.

In order for foods to have longer shelf lives, food companies infuse them with preservatives that inadvertently damage our health. The good news is, once we educate ourselves on what is truly bad for us, we can take easy steps to reduce it in our diets. And this doesn't mean giving up quick and easy eating.

The first step to improving circulation through nutrition is simply knowing the **Bad Stuff** and the **Good Stuff** ... and what makes them good and bad.

The Bad Stuff

While there are many foods that you know to be bad, you might be surprised by some others.

Fried foods, foods high in sodium, foods high in "bad" fat, white bread, white pasta, white rice, foods with refined sugar, high fructose corn syrup, and glucose all cause a variety of blood flow issues.

The Confusion About Fat

It is important to realize that there are good and bad fats. The body needs good fat to be healthy, but bad fat can have profoundly unhealthy consequences.

Foods that contain high amounts of saturated (bad) fat—particularly those high in trans fat—greatly contribute to LDL (bad cholesterol) deposits in the bloodstream. This bad cholesterol is "sticky" and adheres to the sides of arteries, eventually causing reduced blood flow or even complete blockage, which can lead to a heart attack. So prevalent is high cholesterol in our society that, according to health industry data firm IMS Health, more than 255 million prescriptions for lipid regulators (cholesterol-lowering drugs) were filled by pharmacies in 2010.[1]

Sodium – the Silent Killer

One of the most overlooked culprits of poor circulation and health is sodium overload. Most people think that consuming too much salt simply means you get thirsty or your fingers swell, making it hard to get your rings off. Both are true, but understanding *why* your body becomes thirsty and retains water is critical in understanding its effects on circulation.

---

[1] *The Use of Medicines in the United States: Review of 2010*, IMS Institute for Healthcare Informatics.

Why Does Salt Make Us Thirsty?

Sodium is an electrolyte (as is potassium), which carries electrical impulses throughout our body. In order for us to function properly, the concentration of electrolytes in our body must remain consistent.

Increased concentrations of electrolytes in our blood make us thirsty. Why? Because our body is trying to tell us that it needs more water to balance out the high concentration of electrolytes. Why do you think pubs provide bowls of salty snacks? More salt, more thirst, and more drinks sold!

Consuming an adequate amount of water will help our kidneys balance the electrolytes in our blood, and help flush excess retained water.

Retaining less water can also help regulate blood pressure. Water moves beyond our bloodstream, just like other nutrients, feeding our cells, tissues, and organs. Through osmosis, water flows from a lower salinity (salt concentration) to a higher one, attempting to balance the levels. Ever get bloated or feel puffy after eating too much salt? That's water moving from our bloodstream to our body tissue in an attempt to balance things out.

Sodium is directly linked to high blood pressure and poor blood flow, which can lead to heart disease or stroke. And sodium is sneaky, too—there is an alarming amount lurking in foods that you might not consider "salty." Ketchup,

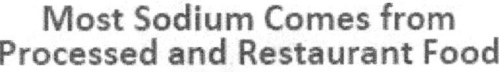

Most Sodium Comes from Processed and Restaurant Food

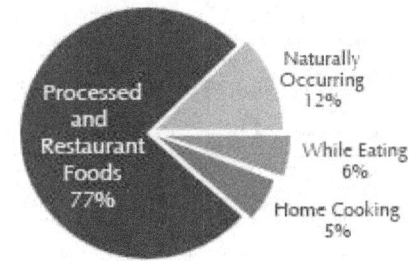

American cheese singles, devil's food cake mix, cottage cheese, packaged meats, canned vegetables—you can find large amounts of sodium in nearly all processed foods.

The Department of Agriculture lists various foods and their sodium content, and many foods may surprise you.

- Dehydrated onion soup mix (1 packet) – 3,132 mg
- Seasoned bread crumbs (1 cup) – 2,111 mg
- Spaghetti sauce (1 cup) – 1,203 mg
- Canned chicken noodle soup (1 cup) – 1,106 mg
- Frozen turkey and gravy (5 ounces) – 787 mg
- Canned cream-style corn (1 cup) – 730 mg
- Teriyaki sauce (1 tablespoon) – 690 mg
- Vegetable juice cocktail (1 cup) – 653 mg
- Canned jalapeno peppers (¼ cup) – 434 mg

Restaurant foods also have high concentrations of sodium. The graph on the previous page shows where the majority of the sodium that we consume comes from.[2]

According to the Center for Disease Control (CDC), for people over 40, African Americans, and those with high blood pressure, the recommended daily allowance of sodium is 1,500 mg. The average American consumes more than *double* that amount (about 3,500 mg) EVERY DAY! The CDC also reports that in 2005/2006, 29% of adults had hypertension (high blood pressure), and an additional 28% had pre-hypertension.[3] That's more than *half the population*!

So the next time you pick up that can of green beans that you thought was so good for you, read the sodium content on the label and pay special attention to the serving size (see Reading Nutrition Labels later in this chapter) to be sure that what you are eating won't put you at risk.

---

[2] Mattes, RD, and D. Donnelly. "Relative contributions of dietary sodium sources." *Journal of the American College of Nutrition* 10, no. 4 (August 1991): 383–393.

[3] *Most Americans Should Consume Less Sodium* (1,500 mg/Day or Less), Center for Disease Control and Prevention, 2011. Application of Lower Sodium Intake Recommendations to Adults - United States, 1999–2006. Reported by: C Ayala, PhD, EV Kuklina, MD, PhD, J Peralez, MPH, NL Keenan, PhD, DR Labarthe, MD, PhD, Div for Heart Disease and Stroke Prevention, National Center for Chronic Disease Prevention and Health Promotion, CDC, http://www.cdc.gov/features/sodium.

Sugar, Sugar Everywhere

If you think the issues with sugar and circulation are limited to weight and diabetes, this information may surprise you.

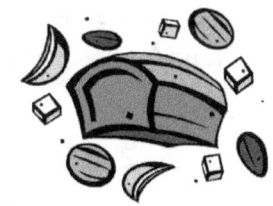

Sugar-sweetened beverages, such as soda and energy drinks, are linked to an increase in high blood pressure. It is thought that this rise in blood pressure levels is a result of an increase in the level of uric acid in the blood, which may in turn lower the nitric oxide required to keep the blood vessels dilated. Sugar consumption has also been linked to enhanced sympathetic nervous system activity and sodium retention.[4]

When we think of foods high in sugar, we tend to think of the obvious—desserts, soda, and candy. But foods high in sugar are all around us. Fruit juice, for example, is often loaded with added sugar. Canned fruit, cereal, and many processed foods are also sugar-laden. And if you've never followed a low-carb diet, you might not realize that foods like white bread, pasta, potatoes, corn, and carrots—all off-limits on a low-carb diet—are high in sugar as well. Although these foods do not contain refined sugar, they turn into sugar in your bloodstream, causing the same effect.

Sugar's connection to health issues is so prevalent, in fact, that the American Heart Association released guidelines to help people understand what a healthy intake of sugar is.[5] For adult women, 5 teaspoons (20 grams) of sugar per day is recommended. For adult men, it's 9 teaspoons (36 grams) daily, and for children, it's only 3 teaspoons (12 grams) a day. Within those same guidelines, it is estimated that the average American adult is consuming more than 22 teaspoons per day,

---

[4] American Heart Association. "Sugar-sweetened drinks associated with higher blood pressure." *ScienceDaily* (March 1, 2011), http://www.sciencedaily.com/releases/2011/02/110228163030.htm (accessed October 14, 2011).

[5] "Dietary Sugars Intake and Cardiovascular Health: A Scientific Statement From the American Heart Association." Rachel K. Johnson, Lawrence J. Appel, Michael Brands, Barbara V. Howard, Michael Lefevre, Robert H. Lustig, Frank Sacks, Lyn M. Steffen and Judith Wylie-Rosett, http://circ.ahajournals.org/content/120/11/1011.full.pdf.

and the average child between 14 and 17 teaspoons per day. It's no wonder obesity is such an epidemic!

Double Doses of Danger

Combining less-than-healthy foods can cause double or triple doses of danger. For instance, a lunch consisting of a lunchmeat ham sandwich on white bread with regular mayonnaise, a slice of American cheese, carrots, and a glass of juice sounds like a pretty healthy meal, right? Not so. This meal contains nearly 30 grams of sugar, 56 grams of carbohydrates, and a whopping 1,287 milligrams of sodium!

But don't get discouraged. Small changes make a big difference. Substituting whole grain bread for white bread, skipping the cheese, switching mustard for regular mayo, low-sodium meat or fresh turkey for ham, celery for carrots and water for juice saves you about 500 milligrams of sodium and 24 grams of sugar, and turns an unhealthy meal into a healthy one.

Top 10 Foods to Avoid

1. Bacon and Other Cured Meats

OK, so this is no big surprise. Bacon has long been known as a diet no-no. But what you might not know is that regular consumption of processed and cured meats like bacon and hot dogs can increase your risk of heart disease by 42%, and diabetes by 19%![6] If I told you that holding an umbrella next to a bus stop would increase your chances of getting hit by a bus by 42%, would you do it? No!

---

[6] "Red and Processed Meat Consumption and Risk of Incident Coronary Heart Disease, Stroke, and Diabetes Mellitus, A Systematic Review and Meta-Analysis." Renata Micha, RD, PhD; Sarah K. Wallace, BA; Dariush Mozaffarian, MD, http://circ.ahajournals.org/content/121/21/2271.abstract.

The reasons bacon and cured meats are so bad is that first of all, they are high in fat. All you need to do is look at a slice of bacon to see how high the fat content is. If you're looking at a slice that is one-half meat and one-half fat, you're lucky. The majority is usually pure fat. Then comes the curing process. Bacon and cured meats are either injected or soaked in a brine solution, or pure salt. In fact, a single slice of bacon can contain over 1,000 milligrams of sodium!

If you absolutely must eat processed meat, make your indulgences few and far between, and follow them up with plenty of water to flush it out of your system as quickly as possible.

> **The Alternative:** *Sorry to say that there really is no "healthy" alternative to bacon and other cured meats—at least none that come close in taste. Your best bet is to just stay away from them as much as you can. But, if you simply cannot go without them, you can try alternatives like turkey bacon, vegetarian bacon, and nitrate-free or low-sodium bacon. Remember, moderation is always the key!*

---

2. Refined Sugar, White Bread & Pasta

Regular consumption of refined sugar (cane sugar and corn syrup), or sugar-producing foods, such as potatoes, white bread, and pasta, can lead to an excess of insulin in your blood, which can cause: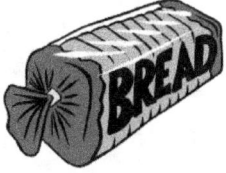

- Increased sodium retention, a known cause of high blood pressure
- Weight gain
- Blood vessel damage and blood clot development through an increased amount of inflammatory compounds in your blood
- An increased risk of heart disease through an increase in triglycerides and LDL (bad cholesterol) and a reduction in HDL (good cholesterol)

- A reduction in magnesium, a mineral that is necessary to keep blood vessels relaxed for proper blood flow

The insulin spikes in your bloodstream can be difficult for your body to regulate. If you or someone you know regularly checks their blood-sugar levels because of diabetes, you know what I mean. The simple act of eating a piece of white bread or a cookie can cause a spike in blood sugar, followed by a dip. A diabetic who dips too far can actually experience a seizure, diabetic coma, or even death.

Even those of us fortunate enough not to have diabetes can feel the effects of blood sugar spikes and drops. Just give a kid a big glass of juice and a slice of birthday cake. When he's done, watch him run around the house like a lunatic for the next 15 minutes … then have a meltdown because he can't find a toy.

Or how about us grown-ups? We'll leave the office for lunch and chow down a burger and some fries. We'll feel full, but pretty good until about 3 p.m. Then, it's all we can do to keep our eyes open in the afternoon meeting!

> **Did You Know...**
>
> People diagnosed with pre-diabetes have a condition in which their blood-glucose levels are higher than normal, but not high enough to be considered diabetes.
>
> Pre-diabetics have a higher risk of being diagnosed with Type 2 diabetes; however, the condition can be improved.
>
> Eating a healthy diet and getting the proper amount of exercise can help return blood glucose levels to normal.

> **The Alternative:** *Luckily, there are many readily available healthy alternatives to refined sugar, white bread, and pasta. The revelation over the past fifteen years or so that refined sugar and white carbs cause blood-sugar spikes and weight gain has opened up a new world of whole grain foods with less sugar.*

Now, without much looking, you can find whole grain bread, pasta, and packaged foods that are either sugar free, no sugar added, or low sugar. Simply replacing white bread and pasta with whole grains will make a big difference!

3. Fried Food

It should come as no surprise that fried food is on our list of foods to avoid. For years, doctors and dieticians have warned us that making fried foods a big part of our diets can lead to weight gain and heart disease. The reason? Fried foods are often cooked in vegetable oil, which contains trans fats. Trans fats increase LDL (bad cholesterol) in our bloodstream and lower HDL (good cholesterol). And as we know, high cholesterol leads to clogged arteries, which lead to heart disease and Type 2 diabetes. And if the high fat and cholesterol content weren't enough, fried foods are generally battered in white flour. This adds to spikes in blood sugar, another cause of arterial stress.

> **The Alternative:** *Oven-baking is a way to get that comfort-food feeling without all the health risks. You can replace traditional white bread crumbs or cornmeal batter with whole wheat bread crumbs or crushed nuts, like pecans. By using egg whites and skim milk in a batter for your fish or chicken, you also cut down on a lot of the cholesterol and fat of traditional deep-fried food.*

4. Carryout Chinese Food

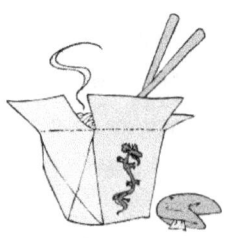

Chinese food, when prepared at your typical American Chinese restaurant, is one of the worst offenders when it comes to heart and circulatory health risks. Yummy as it may be, most Chinese food—even the vegetables—are loaded with fat and sodium.

Many Chinese dishes are breaded and deep-fried, allowing excess fat to soak into the food and end up in your arteries. That fat, combined with an enormous amount of sodium, is by all standards a no-no.

Take your typical plate of General Tso's chicken, for instance. At about 1,300 calories, 11 grams of saturated fat, and 3,200 milligrams of sodium, it contains more than twice the amount of sodium and half the total calories the average adult should consume in one day!

> **The Alternative:** *The best way to enjoy Chinese food is to learn to prepare it at home. Find low-sodium sauces or make your own. Stir-fry your own veggies in olive oil, and be sure your chicken is stir-fried or grilled, not battered and deep-fried. If you have to eat Chinese food out, choose dishes that are likely to have less fat, such as stir-fried chicken and vegetables.*

5. Fast Food

Not a day goes by, it seems, that we don't hear someone warning us of the dangers of fast food. Blamed for child and adult obesity and even death, fast food has long been known as a health risk. Why? Fast food by design must be prepared inexpensively and be able to withstand long-distance shipping. Therefore, fillers, preservatives, and cheap ingredients are the foundation of fast food.

But let's not stop there. How about we drop those cheap ingredients into a vat of saturated fat to heat them up? Then let's put them on white bread, spread ketchup and mayo on them, and serve them up with some fries and a soda. And if we feel like being really, *really* bad, let's top it off with a shake.

If fast food came with nutrition information labels, you may think twice about what you choose. Let's take a look at what you'd be putting into your system if you ordered that naughty menu above.[7].

Food	Calories	Calories From Fat	Total Fat	Trans Fat	Cholesterol	Sodium	Carbs
Big Mac	540	260	29 g	1.5 g	75 mg	1040 mg	45 g
Fries	500	220	25 g	0 g	0 mg	350 mg	63 g
Coke	210	0	0 g	0 g	0 mg	15 mg	58 g
Shake	880	24	37 g	1.5 g	75 mg	370 mg	147 g
Totals	**2130**	**504**	**91 g**	**3 g**	**150 mg**	**1775 mg**	**313 g**

All it takes is one viewing of the documentary *Supersize Me* to truly grasp the very real dangers of fast food. If you're concerned at all about your circulation, do everything you can to avoid fast food.

> ***The Alternative:*** *Fast food may be quick and easy, but there are cheaper, healthier options. We generally choose fast food because it's, well, fast. We're either on the go, or we simply don't have time to cook. Knowing that we have a busy lifestyle and that we may often be in a situation where we need food fast, it's a good idea to keep healthy items on hand that we can either grab or prepare quickly. For instance, keep a few food bars or snacks in your car, along with some bottled water. Granola bars are great, as are re-sealable bags of trail mix or nuts. While that may not be a meal, it's surely enough to tide you over until you can find time to eat something good.*

---

[7] Nutrition facts as published by McDonald's Corporation, http://nutrition.mcdonalds.com/nutritionexchange/nutritionfacts.pdf.

As for lacking time to prepare a meal at home, that too can be taken care of with a little planning. Instead of bringing home a burger, for example, try taking a few slices of whole grain bread, adding some turkey, provolone cheese, tomato, and a smidge of mustard or low-fat mayonnaise and grilling it either on a Panini grill or just on the stove. Serve it up with some veggie chips or a side salad for a very quick, very yummy meal.

6. Donuts, Pies and Pastries

Donuts are not only loaded with refined sugar and white carbs, but are also dunked in oil, deep-fried, and topped with sugar! Pies and pastries also tend to be very high in sugar and refined white flour. And while you might 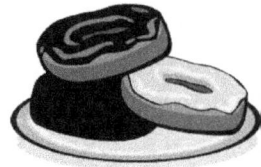 crave them (sugar is addictive), they are not a wise choice for those looking to improve circulation. One chocolate frosted donut, for instance, has 15 grams of fat and 31 grams of carbohydrates.

Food	Calories	Calories from Fat	Total Fat	Saturated Fat	Sugar	Sodium	Carbs
Chocolate Frosted Donut	240	140	15 g	7 g	13 g	340 mg	31 g

The Alternative: Any sort of fruit is a healthier alternative for a sweet craving. A banana, for example, starts off your day with sweetness that won't cause you to crash in the middle of the day, and it has the added benefit of sodium-reducing potassium.

7. Pasta & Potato Salads

Just because it has the word "salad" in it doesn't mean it's good for you! Non-green salads, such as pasta salad and potato salad, can be a high-calorie, high-fat diet-killer. When prepared with white pasta and high-fat sauces like mayonnaise, pasta salads can contain as much as 20 grams of fat or more.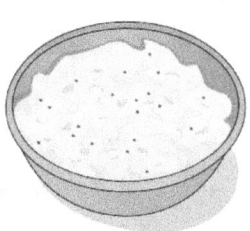

A leading brand of **Bacon Ranch Pasta Salad**, for example, contains 21 grams of fat in a mere ¾-cup serving.

Calories	350	Sodium	510 mg
Total Fat	21 g	Potassium	0 mg
Saturated	3 g	Total Carbs	34 g
Polyunsaturated	0 g	Dietary Fiber	2 g
Monounsaturated	0 g	Sugars	5 g
Trans	0 g	Protein	7 g
Cholesterol	15 mg		

The Alternative: Whole grain pasta is a much healthier alternative to typical white pasta. Also, instead of drenching your pasta in fatty dressings, try using olive oil and natural herbs and spices to give your food flavor.

8. Processed Cheese

While some cheese, consumed in moderation, is good for you, processed cheese like American cheese slices and squirt cheese in a can should be avoided. A single 1-ounce slice of American cheese contains 22% of your recommended daily allowance of saturated fat! And although makers of squirt cheese in a can brag that it is an excellent source of calcium (they add calcium nitrate), it contains no other ingredients that have health benefits. Made with whey (a filler), salt, sodium citrate, sodium phosphate, sodium alginate, and apocarotenal (the ingredient that makes it orange), this food (can we call it a food?) simply fills space in your stomach.

> **The Alternative:** *Real cheese has many health benefits. Cheese is high in calcium, which strengthens bones and helps prevent cavities. Cheese also contains nutrients, such as vitamin A, vitamin B12, zinc, and riboflavin. Cheese can, however, be high in fat and should be consumed in moderation.*

9. Alcohol (in excess)

As we discussed earlier, drinking alcohol in excess can constrict blood vessels and increase your blood pressure, increasing the risk of a heart attack or stroke. That, in addition to the fact that alcohol is a depressant and has mood-altering effects, means that drinking it in excess is something to avoid.

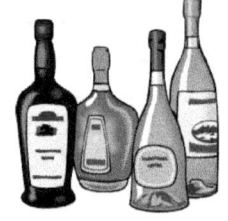

> **The Alternative:** *Drinking alcohol in moderation (one drink per day) can actually dilate the blood vessels, making your heart work less. So, drinking a small amount of alcohol a day will actually help your circulation.*

10. Classic Potato Chips & Snack Foods

Potatoes are a white starch and thus produce sugar in the blood. Add deep-frying and salt to that and you have a snack that's not good for promoting healthy circulation. Other bagged snacks have similar issues: too much starch, too much salt, and too much fat. In just 11 potato chips, for instance, there are 10 grams of fat.

Classic Wavy Potato Chips (11 chips)

Calories	160	Sodium	140 mg
Total Fat	10 g	Potassium	340 mg
Saturated	1 g	Total Carbs	15 g
Polyunsaturated	3 g	Dietary Fiber	1 g
Monounsaturated	5 g	Sugars	0 g
Trans	0 g	Protein	2 g
Cholesterol	0 mg		

Baked Ruffle Potato Chips

Calories	110	Sodium	120 mg
Total Fat	3 g	Potassium	220 mg
Saturated	0 g	Total Carbs	19 g
Polyunsaturated	2 g	Dietary Fiber	2 g
Monounsaturated	1 g	Sugars	1 g
Trans	0 g	Protein	2 g
Cholesterol	0 mg		

The Alternative: *Avoid bagged snacks and opt for snacking on veggies or nuts. If you absolutely must snack, try baked snacks or veggie chips instead. Baked potato chips, while still containing white starch, have far less fat than classic chips.*

The Good Stuff

So we've sufficiently beaten you up about what not to eat. Now, let's focus on the good stuff. Fruits, vegetables, foods high in protein, good fat, complex carbohydrates, and antioxidants work naturally with your body to keep blood oxygenated and vessels and arteries flexible. But you might be surprised at some of the foods that can actually help increase your circulation. There are plenty out there. Here we have picked **10 Foods that Help Increase Circulation** to help get you started!

10 Foods that Help Increase Circulation

1. Cayenne pepper
2. Watermelon
3. Oranges (vitamin C)
4. Garlic
5. Bananas (potassium)
6. Fish (omega-3)
7. Seeds/Nuts (vitamin E)
8. Alcohol (moderate)
9. Apple cider vinegar
10. Cocoa

1. Cayenne Pepper

Eating cayenne pepper and other hot peppers is thought to be one of the most powerful ways to increase your blood flow and metabolic rate. More simply put, it *burns fat*. Put a little cayenne pepper on your tongue and you will instantly feel the increase in blood flow.

As a supplement, cayenne comes in heat units (HU) of 40,000, 60,000, and 90,000, with the highest number having the greatest benefit. Cayenne pepper is thought by many to be a miracle cure for everything from acne to cancer. It has even been reported to instantly stop a heart attack. While that may be a tall tale, cayenne pepper most certainly has circulation benefits.

2. Watermelon

If you're looking for a sweet treat that will increase circulation and get you "in the mood," try watermelon. Watermelon is rich in citrulline, an amino acid that helps increase blood flow to the heart and sex organs. The highest concentration of citrulline is found in the rind of the watermelon; however, there is still enough of it in the flesh to deliver its benefits.

3. Oranges – Vitamin C

Antioxidant-rich vitamin C has many health benefits; one of which is increasing circulation. A study of people with Type 2 diabetes proved that vitamin C increased circulation by improving endothelial cell performance within blood vessels.[8]

People with Type 2 diabetes do not produce or release nitric oxide, an enzyme that adds oxygen to nitrogen in the blood. Endothelial cells—a layer of flat cells lining the interior of blood vessels—rely on the circulation of nitric oxide to function properly. Whether or not you have Type 2 diabetes, you simply cannot go wrong by incorporating vitamin C in your diet.

4. Garlic

Garlic is widely thought to have many health benefits, including helping to manage blood pressure. As we learned in Chapter 1, high blood pressure is damaging to your arteries, and therefore must be kept in check. Adding fresh garlic to food will also help you use less salt, a known contributor to high blood pressure.

5. Bananas – Potassium

Bananas are a great source of potassium, a mineral that blunts the effects of sodium and helps control blood pressure. Other good sources of potassium include cantaloupes, peas, sweet potatoes, tomatoes, honeydew melons, kidney beans, prunes, raisins, and fat-free or 1% milk.

---

[8] "Vitamin C Improves Endothelium-dependent Vasodilation in Patients with Non–Insulin-dependent Diabetes Mellitus" Henry H. Ting, Farris K. Timimi, Kimberly S. Boles, Shelly J. Creager, Peter Ganz, and Mark A. Creager http://www.ncbi.nlm.nih.gov/pmc/articles/PMC507058/pdf/970022.pdf.

6. Fish – Omega 3

Omega-3 fatty acids found in fish have been shown to reduce cholesterol and are currently being prescribed in pill form for patients with high cholesterol. A new study suggests that omega-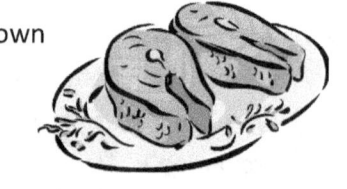
3s from fish are also responsible for lowering the risk of coronary heart disease (CHD).

In fact, a recent study conducted with women in the Nurses' Health Study reported an inverse association between fish intake and omega-3 fatty acids and CHD death. Compared with women who rarely ate fish (less than once per month), the risk of CHD death was 21% lower for those who consumed fish 1–3 times per month; 29% lower for those who consumed fish once per week; 31% lower for those who consumed fish 2–4 times per week; and 34% lower for those who consumed fish 5 times per week.[9]

7. Seeds & Nuts

Seeds like pumpkin seeds and flax seeds, as well as many nuts, are high in vitamin E, which helps stop the production of plaque in your bloodstream and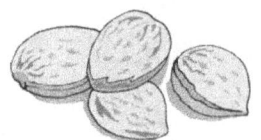
lower cholesterol. Many nuts are good plant-based sources of omega-3s and fiber, both shown to lower cholesterol. The added bonus is that seeds and nuts are readily available, easy to store, and easy to take with you anywhere! For nuts and seeds that come in cans or jars, however, you want to pay special attention to added salt and seasoning, which add unneeded sodium.

---

[9] "Fish and Omega-3 Fatty Acid Intake and Risk of Coronary Heart Disease in Women" Frank B. Hu, Leslie Bronner, Walter C. Willett, Meir J. Stampfer, Kathryn M. Rexrode, Christine M. Albert, David Hunter, JoAnn E. Manson. JAMA. 2002;287(14):1815-1821.http://jama.ama-assn.org/content/287/14/1815.full.pdf+html?sid=e3fa4067-5134-4eea-96cd-0848e6e195d0.

8. Alcohol (moderate)

Although there is much debate about the effects of alcohol on circulation and the heart, all indicators suggest that light to moderate alcohol consumption can be beneficial for some. The issue seems to be *where* the scale tips from beneficial to bad. In a study presented at the American Heart Association's Scientific Session 2010, light to moderate alcohol consumption (about 2 drinks per day) among male coronary artery bypass patients was associated with 25% fewer subsequent cardiovascular procedures, heart attacks, strokes, and death than non-drinkers.[10]

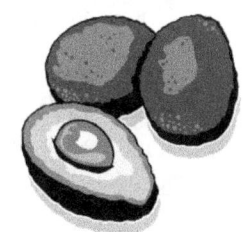

9. Avocados

Avocados are considered by some to be a "super food." They are rich in numerous beneficial nutrients, such as glutathione (antioxidant), carotenoid lutein (eye health), beta-sitosterol (cholesterol health), folate (prevents strokes), and vitamin E. So far-reaching are the benefits of avocados, they may need to change the saying to "An avocado a day keeps the doctor away!"

10. Cocoa

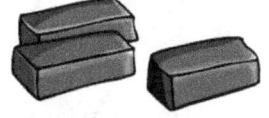

According to the National Confectioners Association Chocolate Council, in various studies over the past five years that examined the cocoa and chocolate eating habits of over 90,000 adults, individuals who ate chocolate on some regular basis were less likely to develop a range of cardiovascular problems. Findings also included a reduction in overall mortality and blood pressure.[11]

---

[10] American Heart Association (2010, November 14). Light to moderate drinking linked to fewer heart problems in male bypass patients, study finds. ScienceDaily. Retrieved November 3, 2011, from http://www.sciencedaily.com- /releases/2010/11/101114161823.htm

[11] "Taking Chocolate to Heart: For Pleasure and Health." National Confectioners Association, http://thestoryofchocolate.com/files/Microsite/TakingChocolateToHeart020311.pdf

Before you reach for that candy bar, though, note that the higher the cocoa content in the chocolate, the greater the benefits. Unprocessed cocoa has the largest amount of antioxidants from flavonoids, which provide the cardiovascular benefits.

Now that we know about some foods that can give us a circulation boost, let's take a look at ways we can regulate our daily consumption of unhealthy food.

Reading Nutrition Labels

Unless you're a dieter or someone who is paying close attention to your health, you may not be an avid nutrition label reader. Nutrition labels are the first place to start when making the decision to improve circulation and live a healthier life. Food manufacturers are required by law to disclose the ingredients they put in their foods and list nutritional values.

To properly read and follow nutrition labels, it's a good idea to know what you're looking for. Once you've learned which parts of the label are most important for good circulatory health, making better choices at the grocery store will be easy!

If nutrition labels look like stereo instructions to you, don't worry. The FDA—regulators of what goes on nutrition labels—offers helpful advice on how to read and interpret these labels. Essentially, a good rule of thumb is ... *the bad stuff is at the top, and the good stuff is at the bottom*!

Here is how the FDA explains how to read nutrition labels[12]:

Sample label for
Macaroni & Cheese

Nutrition Facts

Start Here ➡️ Serving Size 1 cup (228g)
Servings Per Container 2

Check Calories

Amount Per Serving

Calories 250   Calories from Fat 110

	% Daily Value*
Total Fat 12g	18%
Saturated Fat 3g	15%
Trans Fat 3g	
Cholesterol 30mg	10%
Sodium 470mg	20%
Total Carbohydrate 31g	10%
Dietary Fiber 0g	0%
Sugars 5g	
Protein 5g	
Vitamin A	4%
Vitamin C	2%
Calcium	20%
Iron	4%

Limit these Nutrients

Get Enough of these Nutrients

Quick Guide to % DV

_____

• **5% or less is Low**

• **20% or more is High**

* Percent Daily Values are based on a 2,000 calorie diet. Your Daily Values may be higher or lower depending on your calorie needs.

	Calories:	2,000	2,500
Total Fat	Less than	65g	80g
Sat Fat	Less than	20g	25g
Cholesterol	Less than	300mg	300mg
Sodium	Less than	2,400mg	2,400mg
Total Carbohydrate		300g	375g
Dietary Fiber		25g	30g

Footnote

---

[12] http://www.fda.gov/food/labelingnutrition/consumerinformation/ucm078889.htm

When focusing on circulation, pay special attention to **saturated fat**, **cholesterol**, and **sodium**—the items labeled "Limit these Nutrients" on the guide above. It's important to pay attention to it all, but those are the three easiest ones to start with. After that, take a look at carbohydrates, sugars, fiber, and protein, and be sure that nothing looks too out of whack. Limit your intake of carbohydrates that do not contain dietary fiber, and pay added attention to sugar.

Let's take a look at what's recommended. For adults eating 2,000 calories per day, the DRVs (daily recommended values) are:

Total Fat	65 g
Saturated Fatty Acids	20 g
Cholesterol	300 mg
Sodium	2300 mg
Potassium	4700 mg
Total Carbohydrates	300 g
Fiber	25 g
Protein	50 g

What's Your Daily Intake?

To see how you're doing, try spending just one day eating what you would normally eat and write down your nutrition intake. This is tough when eating out, so choose a day when you will be eating foods from the store, where nutrition labels are available.

When logging your intake, be honest not only about the nutrition information, but also your portion size. Makers of foods high in all the wrong ingredients are notorious for including small portion sizes on their nutrition labels. Who eats a half cup of cereal? If your portion size is larger than what's listed on the nutrition label, do the math and figure out exactly what you're taking in.

CIRCULATION PURIFICATION

A good first step in preparing your body for lifestyle changes and achieving Circulation Domination! is Circulation Purification.

Recently, the body detox craze has taken off. Often used to kick-start a weight loss program, body detoxing is a way to rid cells of toxins that can cause us to feel sluggish or even cause illness.

Toxins are anything that can harm our body tissue. These toxins include normal cell waste—waste that is a result of normal cell activity—like ammonia, lactic acid, and homocysteine, an amino acid produced by the body that is generally a by-product of red meat. It also includes environmental toxins, such as cigarette smoke, pesticides, household cleaners, food additives and drugs, which come from our air, food, and water.

Naturally, our intestines, kidneys, liver, lungs, skin, blood, and lymphatic systems work hand-in-hand to rid our bodies of these toxins. When these systems are not performing at their best, however, toxins can build up. Increased levels of toxins like homocysteine, for example, can cause atherosclerosis (hardening and narrowing of the arteries), as well as an increased risk of heart attack, stroke, and blood clot formation.

So, the first step in our action plan for achieving *Circulation Domination!* is to focus on purification. There is a lot of buzz about over-the-counter detox and cleanse programs, which do a good job cleaning out your colon temporarily. Whether or not they truly rid cells of toxins is up for debate.

The best way to purify your system is to embark on a cleansing diet. Elements of a cleansing diet include:

- Plenty of water, but not too much (6–8 glasses per day should suffice), and high-fiber foods to help flush out your system through urination and bowel movements.
- Avoiding foods high in chemicals, such as packaged foods. Organic, fresh food will contain the least amount of chemicals.
- Seeking out foods high in antioxidants (see Top 20 Antioxidant Foods on the following page), vitamins, and essential nutrients.

Couple your cleansing diet with added exercise, and you will be well on your way to Circulation Purification!

Top Antioxidant Foods

Food rich in antioxidants has been shown to help rid the body of harmful toxins. Following is a list of the **Top 20 Antioxidant Foods** as published in the *Journal of Agricultural and Food Chemistry* by the USDA. It is the largest USDA study of food antioxidants[1] and was conducted utilizing updated technology to assess the antioxidant content of more than 100 foods, including fruits, vegetables, cereals, breads, nuts, and spices.

---

[1] American Chemical Society (2004, June 17). Largest USDA Study Of Food Antioxidants Reveals Best Sources. ScienceDaily. Retrieved November 3, 2011, from http://www.sciencedaily.com-/releases/2004/06/040617080908.htm

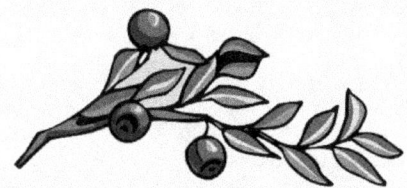

Top 20 Antioxidant Foods

Rank	Food item	Serving Size	Antioxidant capacity per serving size
1.	Small red bean (dried)	½ cup	13727
2.	Wild blueberry	1 cup	13427
3.	Red kidney bean (dried)	½ cup	13259
4.	Pinto bean	½ cup	11864
5.	Blueberry (cultivated)	1 cup	9019
6.	Cranberry	1 cup (whole)	8983
7.	Artichoke (cooked)	1 cup (hearts)	7904
8.	Blackberry	1 cup	7701
9.	Dried prune	½ cup	7291
10.	Raspberry	1 cup	6058
11.	Strawberry	1 cup	5938
12.	Red Delicious apple	One	5900
13.	Granny Smith apple	One	5381
14.	Pecan	1 ounce	5095
15.	Sweet cherry	1 cup	4873
16.	Black plum	One	4844
17.	Russet potato (cooked)	One	4649
18.	Black bean (dried)	½ cup	4181
19.	Plum	One	4118
20.	Gala apple	One	3903

CIRCULATION ACTIVATION!

We have opportunities throughout the day to activate our circulatory system. Get started by using these quick tips for Circulation Activation morning, noon, and night.

In Chapter 4, did you determine that your circulatory system may need some work? Or maybe you are in good shape, but want to maximize your circulation potential to feel and look your very best. It's time for *Circulation Activation*!

Little Steps. Big Results.

By approaching each day as an opportunity to improve your circulation, you will find that taking little steps will yield big results. Before long, these steps will simply become a part of your life—you won't even have to think about them!

To make it easy, the following pages contain some quick tips for incorporating circulation improvement into your everyday routine.

Morning Activation

Rise and shine! It's time to stimulate your mind and body. Your morning routine is the ideal time to get your blood moving and energize your day.

Wake Up

To help get your body working in the morning, keep a bottle or glass of water near your bed. As soon as you wake up, begin sipping water to help your body rehydrate. After all, you've been sleeping for 6–8 hours or more—your body (and blood) is thirsty! During sleep your body can lose one or more pounds of water through respiration and perspiration. Because about 55% of your blood is plasma, and plasma is about 90% water, dehydration can mean a reduction in blood flow by reducing the water content in your blood. Drinking water when you awaken is a quick and easy way to rehydrate and get your blood flowing!

Warm Up

Your morning shower is the perfect time to stimulate your circulation. If you've ever dipped your foot into a hot tub, you know that your skin will instantly become flush with blood flow. And while a cold shower will certainly shock you into alertness, in the long run the vascular constriction that occurs when your body is cold will decrease your blood flow and your energy. To get blood moving freely in the morning, take a nice warm shower.

And if you're looking for an added boost to even the smallest of capillaries, try exfoliating skin with a horsehair brush. While your skin is warm and wet, use a wet horsehair body brush to stimulate blood flow. Start with your feet, brushing upward on your skin with short strokes. Move to your torso, arms, back, and chest. This process not only feels great and exfoliates dead skin, it also gets blood moving all the way up to the largest organ of your body—your skin.

Energize

In the morning, your body has had several hours to rest and digest, and is ready for a new day. We've all heard that breakfast is the most important meal of the day. Why? Because it's our first opportunity to do the right thing nutritionally and set the tone for the rest of our day. We can either stuff ourselves with fat and sugar, or we can energize ourselves with proteins, whole grains, and fruit.

In Chapter 2 we learned that fat and sugar, when consumed regularly or in excess, can have serious effects on blood flow. We also learned of some foods that can actually stimulate an increase in blood flow. When choosing what to eat for your most important meal of the day, choose circulation-stimulating foods and you'll be on your way to a high-energy day!

Daytime Activation

We're up and at 'em, and ready to take on the world! Whether it's off to work, school, or a day of errands, childcare and housework, keeping your body moving is a must.

Opt to Walk

One small step that will add up to many steps (and even miles) is opting to walk. How many times have we circled the parking lot anxiously hoping a driver will vacate that primo spot near the front of the building? Or worse yet, pulled right up to the front and switched on the flashers so we can "just run in real quick." The next time you reach your intended destination, make it a point to park a good distance away. The walk, however brief, adds much needed movement that helps get your blood moving.

Make Moving a Priority

Many of us spend countless hours sitting—sitting at our desks, sitting in our cars, sitting on the couch. If more hours of your day are spent sitting than moving, make it a point to get up and move. For 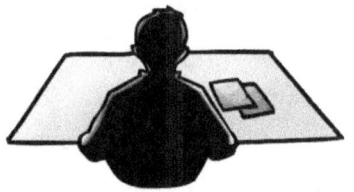 example, if you have a desk job, take a break at least once each hour to get up and walk. If you have stairs nearby, a great way to stimulate your circulation (and even your brain) is doing a few quick flights up and down the steps. You don't have to break a sweat—just a few minutes of walking or stair-climbing can go a long way in increasing blood flow.

Nighttime Activation

Good circulation at night while at rest or asleep is just as important as good circulation when we are up and about. The simple act of eating right, exercising, and staying well-hydrated during the day will already improve our circulation at night.

Other things you can do to improve nighttime circulation include:

Remove Hindrances

If you have ever woken up to an arm or leg being asleep, you know that sleeping in the wrong position or wearing sleep clothes that are too tight can hinder circulation. What you sleep *in* and what you sleep *on* are either helping or hurting circulation.

Wear loose-fitting clothes, and remove rings and other jewelry. Choose a mattress and pillow that offer comfort and proper positioning of your body for maximum blood flow.

Get Solid Sleep

As busy adults in a technology-driven world, we as a society sleep too little. Constant brain stimulation by computers, televisions, and music devices during the day, and a schedule that has us up too early and out too late, results in short sleep durations.

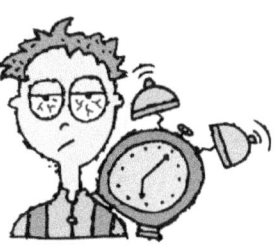

Beyond making us feel tired, sluggish, and unmotivated, there are far worse consequences to a consistent lack of rest. Short sleep duration is linked with:

- Increased risk of motor vehicle accidents.
- A greater likelihood of obesity due to an increased appetite caused by sleep deprivation.
- Increased risk of diabetes and heart problems.
- Increased risk of depression and substance abuse.
- Decreased ability to pay attention, react to signals, or remember new information.

When we wake up each day well-rested, we are more likely to stay on a healthy, happy track. Good sleep is simply imperative for good health, so by all means, make getting a good night's sleep a priority!

CIRCULATION ACCELERATION

Your circulatory system is awake—good job! Don't stop there—make good circulation a part of your daily life. It's time to take it a little further with Circulation Acceleration! We'll cover hydration, nutrition, and physical activity, including a section with circulation-boosting exercises.

To help accelerate your circulation, we'll focus on three main areas:

- Hydration
- Nutrition
- Physical Activity

Hydration

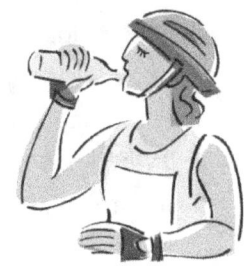

As we mention throughout the book, it is important to keep yourself properly hydrated. The health benefits of drinking water go on and on, but here are just a few:

- Water aids in the digestion of food, allowing it to carry nutrients to the bloodstream.

- Water helps digested food move through and out of the body quicker, preventing toxin and waste buildup.
- Water aids in the metabolism and elimination of fats.
- Water helps rid the body of retained water, often caused by an overconsumption of sodium.
- Water helps regulate body temperature.
- Water is necessary for proper organ function.
- Water keeps our joints, eyes, and skin hydrated and healthy.
- Water aids in brain function.
- Water aids in circulation!

Begin each day with at least one glass of water, and continue to drink water throughout the day. Be sure to consume extra water if you sweat or consume too much sodium. And always drink water when you're thirsty! If water is "boring" to you, jazz it up with some fruit slices, a low-calorie sweetener, or drink decaffeinated tea. Water in its purest form is best, but it's okay to add a bit of flavor if that's what it takes to get you to stay hydrated!

Nutrition

We are what we eat. And, unfortunately, most of us eat poorly. It's not entirely our fault. The introduction of pre-packaged, processed food in the 1950s brought with it the beginning of poor nutrition. Simply putting food in a plastic wrapper isn't enough to keep it from spoiling. Additives, preservatives, fillers, colors, and who knows what else is all added for looks, flavor, and a longer shelf life.

The answer to better nutrition for circulation health is, first and foremost, education—which you now have—and a concerted effort to eat fresh fruits, vegetables, and meats, and cook homemade meals whenever possible. After all, when you fix it, you know exactly what's in it!

Keep the lists we outline in this book (see Chapter 5, "Circulation Nutrition") in mind, and work them into your daily diet:

- **Top 10 Foods to Avoid** *(page 40)*
- **Top 10 Foods that Increase Circulation** *(page 50)*
- **Top 20 Antioxidant Foods** *(page 59)*

Vitamins

In Chapter 5 we learned which foods are good and which are bad. And believe it or not, just knowing is more than half the battle. Armed with knowledge, you can now make healthier choices every day.

To get your circulatory system in good shape, consuming vital nutrients is essential. Although our bodies receive nutrients from the food we eat, it often isn't enough to give us all the essential vitamins we need. In many cases, a daily multivitamin is recommended to help us achieve the proper intake of nutrients.

Physiologically, each human being is as unique as their thumb print. What your body needs to thrive is different from what another person's may need. An annual physical (that includes blood work) by your doctor can help determine where you may be deficient. Some common vitamin deficiencies include vitamin D (needed for healthy bones), vitamin B-12 (needed for proper liver function), calcium and magnesium (both needed for bone health), and iron (needed for energy and proper oxygen transport).

When choosing vitamins, look for those that derive their nutrients from whole foods rather than synthetics. Why? Our bodies are designed to absorb nutrients from the foods we eat. While synthetic vitamins may show a high concentration of nutrients on the label, their absorption rate may be low, and a good portion of those nutrients could pass right through our body without ever being used.

Eating Healthy

Having read many health and fitness books, one of my pet peeves when it comes to nutrition recommendations is unrealistic menus—a month's worth of meals that will have you 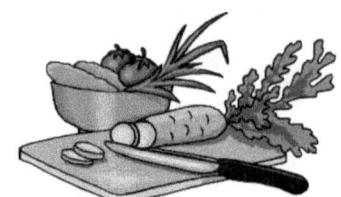 shopping for obscure spices and spending 3 times your normal amount on groceries. Been there. Done that. The result? About a week of sticking to it, then falling right back into old habits. I won't do that here, because I want you to succeed!

Your best bet when it comes to healthy eating is to review the list of good and bad foods in this book, and work on creating your own healthy menu options. Only you know what you like, and what you're likely to fix on a regular basis. The key to sticking with this is to make it a part of your everyday life, not something you try for a week and give up on.

In addition to choosing the healthy food options that suit you best, there are a few rules that I like to follow for healthy eating:

Eat When You are Hungry

Many of us are creatures of habit. We eat at predetermined meal times, whether we are hungry or not. Learn to listen to your body, and when it's hungry, feed it with healthy food.

Eat All Day

Instead of loading up with 3 big meals, eat smaller portions and eat them throughout the day. If you follow the "eat when you are hungry" rule above, you will find that your body functions well and stays energized when you are able to consume smaller portions more often.

Follow the Protein—Carbs—Protein Rule

Begin your day with a protein meal along with some fruit. Many of our breakfast options involve starch—cereal, toast, bagels—but consuming too many carbs at the beginning of your day can spike blood sugar, and by midmorning you're sleepy already! Eggs, cheese, yogurt, and nuts are good protein options. Although meat is high in protein, the harmful elements of breakfast meats like bacon and sausage far outweigh the protein benefits. If you do choose to eat breakfast meat, look for lower fat, lower sodium options.

Eat energy-producing carbohydrates, fruits, and vegetables during the most active part of your day. When you are the most active, your body needs the energy in complex carbohydrates to function efficiently. Although carbohydrates can increase blood sugar, the fact that you are actively working them off lessens the likelihood of blood sugar spikes. The fruits and vegetables will give you added energy and vital nutrients.

End your day with protein and veggies. At night, your body at rest is working to recuperate from the wear and tear of the day. Muscles and cells are rebuilding and need protein and vitamins to do so.

Physical Activity

Every concept outlined in this book for increasing circulation is important, but physical activity is at the top of the list. Living a sedentary lifestyle—no matter what other good things you are doing—is simply bad for your circulation and overall health.

The Centers for Disease Control and Prevention offer guidelines for maintaining a healthy lifestyle that includes physical activity.[1]

---

[1] "How much physical activity do you need?" Centers for Disease Control and Prevention, http://www.cdc.gov/physicalactivity/everyone/guidelines/index.html

For adults ages 18-64, the following is recommended:

2 hours and 30 minutes (150 minutes) of moderate-intensity aerobic activity (e.g., brisk walking) every week and muscle-strengthening activities that work all major muscle groups (legs, hips, back, abdomen, chest, shoulders, and arms) on 2 or more days a week;

OR 1 hour and 15 minutes (75 minutes) of vigorous-intensity aerobic activity (e.g., jogging or running) every week and muscle-strengthening activities that work all major muscle groups on 2 or more days a week;

OR an equivalent mix of moderate- and vigorous-intensity aerobic activity and muscle-strengthening activities that work all major muscle groups on 2 or more days a week.

Does 150 minutes seem daunting? Break it up! If you have 10 minutes or so to spare twice a day (and I know you do!), devote it to cardio activity. You'll work that 150 minutes in with no problem!

Hear What a Fitness Pro Has to Say

Certified fitness instructor and owner of PIOMA Performance Fitness Janice Long provides advice and shares a personal story in this chapter on improving circulation through various yoga and Pilates techniques.

Fitness Instructor Janice Long Shares a Circulation Success Story

"For the past 4½ years, I have been working with Roy, one of the most dedicated Pilates clients I have seen. He is 73 years old. When he came to us, his posture was 'hunched over'—very similar to what I see in many people of his age group.

"As we age, our balance can be compromised, leaving us with a fear of falling. And rightfully so, the response to the body's desire to protect itself is looking down. We want to be more surefooted, so we watch where we are stepping to avoid a potentially damaging fall. The eyes lead the body, and the act of looking down has the effect of drawing the spine into forward flexion (bringing the chest and pelvis closer together).

"The result is a rounding of the shoulders, a head that is forward of the spine (kyphosis), tightened chest muscles, shortened abdominal muscles, and overworked back muscles. This 'hunched over' forward posture greatly reduces not only the capacity of the chest cavity but also the depth of breathing. Therefore, it has a direct impact on the quality and function of oxygenation and gases exchanged in the lungs.

"When I first began working with Roy, it was necessary to place two thick, rolled-up mats under his head when he was lying on the floor or on the Pilates reformer. Even his posture in supine (lying down) was very stressful, much like a turtle on its back. It really wasn't pleasant for him to lie back without something very substantial under his head.

"Roy could only breathe in for a maximum of 2.5 counts during what we call 'the hundred.' The hundred requires a 5-count inhale followed by a 5-count exhale for maximum respiratory and circulatory benefits. A program consisting of simple stretching and breathing exercises was created for Roy, and he can now lie on his back comfortably with nothing under his head. He takes such long, deep breaths that I now count slower than I normally would with other clients. Using a combination of exercise modalities, my 73-year-old client has significantly improved posture, increased lung capacity, and has more solid balance."

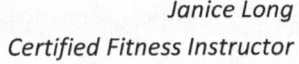

Janice Long
Certified Fitness Instructor

Janice notes that the diversity of training options for improving circulation and achieving fitness goals has improved greatly in recent years. For each client, Janice chooses movements from a vast arsenal for basic strength training, cardiovascular training, flexibility, and overall functional movement. Each is designed to improve the way we move and breathe, to make us stronger, and to improve circulation.

Three exercise methods in particular have, without fail, produced the greatest benefits for Janice's clients without the physical trauma that some training methods can inflict. These modalities include Pilates, yoga, and the Feldenkrais Method®.

Outlined on the following pages are significantly useful exercises for the overall improvement of circulation and health. As with any fitness regimen, it is recommended that you work with a fitness professional to help ensure that you are doing the exercises properly, and that they fit your individual fitness capabilities.

Exercises that Promote Circulation

There are many ways to enhance circulation through physical activity. As you will see, these techniques can be done at any age and can be modified to fit your individual physical capabilities.

Cardiorespiratory Exercises

Cardiorespiratory exercises, otherwise known as aerobic exercises, use large muscle groups and a high level of activity to increase circulation by increasing the heart rate. The more aerobically fit you are, the more blood and oxygen your heart will pump with each beat. Additionally, your muscles will consume more oxygen. The muscles of distance runners, for example, can consume oxygen as much as three times more efficiently than the muscles of someone who gets little to no aerobic exercise.

Ideal cardiorespiratory activities include walking, running, biking, swimming, and even dancing. During these activities, the heart propels blood throughout the body at a greater rate than when at rest, while also distributing blood to areas that may not otherwise get good, consistent circulation.

Walking

For many people, one of the easiest ways to start increasing their level of physical activity is walking. Walking can be done indoors or out, and can be as light or as intense as we make it. Not only is walking an easy way to add movement and get your blood pumping, it can also be good for your mental health and relationships.

Walking alone with no headphones or cell phone gives you time to think clearly—ponder life, solve problems, enjoy nature, whatever you need to reduce stress and clear your head. Walking with a friend or loved one gives you time to talk, away from the distractions of work or home.

Walking has a myriad of other benefits as well. Rodale Inc., the publisher of *Prevention* magazine, *Men's Health* magazine, *Women's Health* magazine, and a host of other health and fitness publications, cited the following *8 Astonishing Benefits of Walking*[2]:

- Reduction in the risk of developing Type 2 diabetes
- Increased sexual desire in women
- Saving money on gym costs

---

[2] Leah Zerbe, "8 Astonishing Benefits of Walking," Rodale.com, June 1, 2010 (last updated May 17, 2011), http://www.rodale.com/benefits-walking.

- Decreased need for medication
- Decreased fibromyalgia pain
- Helps beat breast cancer
- Reduces stroke risk
- Reduces risk of developing dementia

No matter what your age or fitness level, walking is a great way to increase your cardiorespiratory activity.

Running

Nothing gets your heart pumping quite like running! If you are not a runner but are interested in giving it a try, here are a few tips for getting started:

- Talk to your doctor. Before beginning any type of intense activity, it's a good idea to run it by your physician. Depending on your age and current fitness level, your doctor may want to perform a routine physical and advise you how to best get started.
- Invest in proper running shoes. Running can be tough on your feet, knees, hips, and back. To help alleviate any added impact and avoid injury, it's wise to invest in a good pair of shoes specifically designed for running.
- Be sure to eat and drink before running, but not too close to your running time. Your body's ability to get the most out of your aerobic workout relies on it being well-nourished and hydrated. However, consuming food too close to your run may cause stomach cramps or a "side stitch." Although experts are not certain what causes those nasty little pains in your side that can come when you run, many believe it is related to consuming food too close to your run time.

- Take time to stretch and warm up before your run, and stretch and cool down at the end of your run. Avoiding cramps and injuries when running is best accomplished by taking the time to properly stretch your muscles, warm up, and cool down.
- Start off slow and work your way up. Instead of jumping headfirst (or *feet*-first) into running marathons, set some realistic goals. After all, when it comes to fitness, nothing is more discouraging than feeling you failed because you didn't accomplish your goals.
- Keep it interesting. For some, running can be boring. To help keep it interesting, periodically change your surroundings, run with a friend, or run to music.

Biking

Biking (or cycling) is an excellent low-impact form of cardiorespiratory exercise. If you live in an area with bike-friendly streets or bike paths, it is a great way to get outside and get some fresh air and sunshine as well. If you're a city dweller, or live an area that isn't so bike-friendly, you can still enjoy the health benefits of cycling at your local gym, or even in your home with a cycle machine.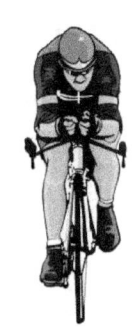

Biking, much like running, increases your heart rate by working your largest muscle groups, found in your thighs. Unlike running, however, biking allows you to work these muscles without high impact. If you have issues with your feet, ankles, knees or hips, biking can be a great alternative to running for high-intensity workouts.

Swimming

Swimming is one of the best ways to get fit. In order to swim, you must use a wide variety of muscle groups in both your upper and lower body. You are required to move constantly, stretching, kicking, and controlling your breathing, making it an excellent way to get your heart pumping.

Swimming is also the lowest impact way to get a good cardio workout. No wonder swimming is often used in physical therapy and rehabilitation!

If you aren't one of the lucky ones who happens to have a pool in their backyard, chances are there is one nearby. Fitness facilities, school campuses, senior centers, and even some hospitals have pools that may be used by the general public. If you are looking to add swimming to your regular fitness routine, check around for public-use pools near you.

Dancing

Nothing provides more fun during a workout (for me, anyway) than putting on some music and just dancing! Upbeat music can lift your mood and make you want to move. Have you ever played music around an infant or toddler and seen them start bouncing or rocking? I'm not sure if you could call it instinctual, but we sure seem to be wired to dance.

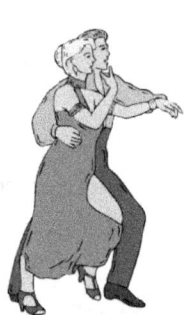

No matter your taste in music, chances are you can dance to it in a way that has fitness benefits. Whether you're waltzing to Mozart, dancing an Irish jig, or busting some hip-hop moves, dancing will get you and your heart rate up!

The key to making cardiorespiratory exercise work for you is to find activities that you truly enjoy.

Breathing Exercises

Proper breathing is essential for good circulatory health. Aside from being aware of *how* we breathe, there are many exercises that can help increase lung capacity.

Yoga

Yoga can be very gentle and restorative in nature or strenuous and vigorous. Most often both ends of the spectrum are achieved in a well-balanced yoga practice. Gravity is a constant force throughout our stress-ridden days of sitting at computers, commuting, and living in a "forward flexed" posture for most of our waking hours.

Yoga Extension Exercises

Throughout our stress-ridden days of sitting at computers, in meetings or in a car, we live in a "forward flexed" posture for most of our waking hours. Yoga poses that promote extension of the spine are fabulous for improving posture, defying the daily impact of gravity on our erectness, and improving circulation. A few basic extension poses help to defy these forces and aid in obtaining a neutral spine. A neutral spine allows for maximum capacity in the lungs, proper functional movement of the spine in all directions—forward flexion, extension, rotation, lateral flexion—and complex combinations of all these healthy movements of the spine.

The following yoga positions can help with breathing, lung capacity, and circulation.

Upward Facing Dog – Upward Facing Dog is a yoga pose designed to stretch your chest and allow for deeper breathing.

Lie facedown on the floor. Stretch your legs back, with the tops of your feet on the floor. Bend your elbows and spread your palms on the floor near your waist, with your forearms perpendicular to the floor.

Inhale and press your hands firmly into the floor, straighten your arms, and simultaneously lift your torso up. If you can, lift high enough so that your legs are a few inches off the floor on a single inhalation. Keep your thighs firm and slightly turned inward. Keep your arms firm and turned out so the elbow creases face forward.

Firm the shoulder blades against the back and gently push the side ribs forward. Avoid pushing the front ribs forward, so as not to harden the lower back. Look straight ahead or tip the head back slightly, but be careful not to harden the throat or back of the neck.

Hold this pose from 15 to 30 seconds, breathing easily. Release back to the floor and exhale.

Sphinx – Lie facedown on your belly with your legs side by side, the tops of your feet on the floor, and your arms at your sides. Buttocks should be firm but not clenched.

Place your elbows under your shoulders and your forearms on the floor parallel to each other. Inhale and lift your upper torso and head away from the floor into a mild backbend. This pose helps with breathing by bringing awareness to your lower belly, just below the navel. Lightly draw it away from the floor, rounding it up toward your lower back. This should be a gentle lift—no hardening—soothing your lower back and awakening your upper back.

Stay in this position for 5 to 10 breaths. Slowly exhale and release your belly. Lower your torso and head to the floor, turning your head to one side. Lie quietly, allowing yourself to exhale and broaden your back, releasing tension with each exhale. Repeat up to 3 times.

Kneeling Back Arch – The kneeling back arch is designed to help with deep breathing.

Sit on the floor on your knees. Press the palms of your hands together near your chest and extend them to the sky. Lift your chest toward the sky, looking up. Take several deep, slow breaths in and out.

Extended Mountain Pose – Another pose designed for deep breathing.

Stand with your feet together firmly on the floor, careful not to lock your knees. Press the palms of your hands together at the chest. Lift your hands toward the sky, looking up. Take several deep, slow breaths in and out.

Yoga Flexion Exercises

Yoga poses that target expansion of the chest and ribs are ideal for promoting increased lung capacity. As we have learned, increasing the quality and quantity of breathing also enhances the overall circulatory benefits.

Child Pose – Kneel on the floor and place your forehead on the floor, chest resting on thighs, hips and tailbone back toward feet.

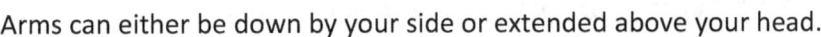

Arms can either be down by your side or extended above your head.

Over a period of 30 seconds to several minutes, take a series of deep breaths. You will notice that—due to the restriction of the abdomen being compressed onto the thighs—the breath is redirected into the back. The ribs will expand, stretching the intercostal muscles between each rib. This is a very strategic way to increase lung capacity by stretching from the inside out.

Pilates Exercise

Pilates provides many benefits for stretching and toning muscles and increasing blood flow. It also assists with breathing. Janice's Pilates exercise of choice for promoting breathing is "the hundred."

The Hundred – This is considered a "warm-up" exercise (but it's so much more!) Lie on your back with your knees bent, feet flat on the floor. Reach your arms toward the ceiling while taking a nice, deep inhale. Exhale while lifting your head and bringing your arms down past the hips. Stay in this position and begin to pump your arms a few inches up and down while keeping the elbows locked and the arms lengthened ("slapping water" is often a useful cue.) Inhale through your nose for 5 counts; exhale through the back of your throat with a "hah" breath for 5 counts (your exhale should be audible, as if you're saying "hah.") Repeat 10 times.

You have just taken in one hundred counts of breath while increasing circulation and taking that wonderful oxygen-rich blood throughout your body in prep for your next exercise.

Everyday Physical Activities

Each of us has the opportunity to help increase our circulation simply by making a conscious effort to move a little more each day. Some easy ideas for increasing your daily movement include:

- *Park a little farther.* At work, the grocery store, school—wherever you go, instead of circling the parking lot like a buzzard hoping for the up-front spot, park a little farther away and walk.

- *Take the stairs.* When given the option to take the elevator or stairs, opt for the stairs, even if it's only for a flight or two.

- *Take movement breaks at work.* If you spend most of your workday behind a desk, make it a point to get up and walk at least once an hour. Kill two birds with one stone and walk to the water fountain for some movement and hydration!

- *Get out and about.* Make plans to get out of the house. Walk a nature trail. Walk the mall. Take a trip into the city and do some sightseeing. Simply getting out and going somewhere will naturally increase your movement and get that blood flowing.

- *Try the treadmill.* Using a treadmill is a great way to add miles of walking to your day, regardless of the weather. Why not take 30–60 minutes of your daily TV time to walk while you watch!

- *Move any way you can.* If you are unable to walk due to age, weight, injury, or other conditions, try to find other ways to move. Pedaling a small stationary wheel with your arms or your legs, for example, will get your muscles and blood flow moving in the right direction.

The One Minute Workout

Who doesn't have 3 minutes a day to devote to improving circulation? To get your blood flowing, try taking just one minute, three times a day to do a cardio-boosting activity. At the beginning, middle, and end of each day, try either running in place, doing jumping jacks, walking or running up and down stairs—whatever gets you moving. I like to mix it up—a little running, a few jumping jacks, and even a little bit of kickboxing gets my heart rate up and my blood pumping. As with any cardio activity, start off slowly, then increase to your max, then take it back down slowly. Everyone's fitness level varies, so only do what you're capable of. Be careful not to take your heart rate too high without taking an adequate amount of time to bring it back down slowly. No matter where you are on the fitness scale, your one-minute workout will improve day by day!

The Fitness Flex

The simple act of flexing or tensing your muscles stimulates additional blood flow. As the muscles contract, arterial blood flow temporarily decreases as the arteries are compressed by the flexing muscle tissue. When the muscles relax, blood flow then increases. Done repeatedly, blood flow is improved to the working muscle.

So even sitting on your couch or at your desk, you have an opportunity to increase blood flow. Throughout the day, just flex! Flex your leg muscles, your arm muscles, tighten your stomach—any muscle that is tensed signals for additional blood flow.

The Weekly Personal Challenge

Let's face it: we all could step up our game every once in a while. As a part of your personal quest for *Circulation Domination!* give yourself some personal challenges. Step it up a notch!

At least once each week, pick a day when you're feeling good and make the conscious decision to take on a new challenge. If you're a walker, try adding a little jogging to the day's walk. If you work on the fifth floor, take the full flight of stairs up to work in the morning. If you normally don't do anything at all, do *something*! You get the idea.

Meeting personal challenges each week will improve your circulation and overall health, and the sense of accomplishment will help your mental well-being.

Just Breathe

Most of us take breathing for granted. It's just something we do. But as we learned in Chapter 2, most of us are only utilizing a portion of our lungs. And in order to properly oxygenate blood, we should be doing much more.

Follow the steps outlined in Chapter 2 for improving your lung capacity and daily oxygen intake. When you do, you will soon feel the benefits.

I certainly did. After several years of a regimented fitness program, I decided to push myself a little more and started running. My previous workout routine was somewhat rigorous and included high-intensity cardio workouts, weights, and stretching. It wasn't until I began running, however, that I began to pay close attention to my breathing.

As a kid, I suffered from exercise-induced asthma. I could never really run long distances or play as hard as the other kids without feeling as if I was trying to breathe under water. Back then, my solution was simply to not run! But as an adult making a concerted effort to be fit, I decided to challenge myself and give it a solid try.

In the beginning it was tough. It felt like no matter how much I tried, I couldn't get enough air to keep me going. It was then that I started making breathing exercises a part of my daily routine. Now I begin and end each day with deep-breathing exercises. And during the day, whenever I think about it, I practice deep breathing.

I also make sure that I am well-hydrated and well-nourished before doing any type of high-intensity workout. There is definitely a difference in my ability to breathe and my stamina when I haven't taken in enough food energy and water.

The result of these efforts was a nearly instant increase in my running stamina. My breathing is less labored; I can run farther; and instead of feeling drained and tired after working out, I feel energized!

CIRCULATION RETENTION

Circulation Domination! is not a fad or a quick fix for what ails you. Circulation Domination! is a way of life that will improve your health and well-being, now and for the rest of your life.

Half the battle of achieving good health is education. Hopefully this book has opened your eyes to the importance of good circulation, and how making simple changes can make a big difference. And now that we know, it's time we retain that knowledge and make it a part of our lives. It's time for *Circulation Retention*.

As with any program that you wish to make a part of your life for self-improvement, I suggest starting with a strong mental commitment, then tracking your goals and progress. I'm a big fan of writing things down. Somehow putting pen to paper (or fingers to keyboard) makes my mental commitment final. Also, having something written down in front of me helps me remember to do it.

So I suggest that your journey to *Circulation Domination!* begin with some soul-searching to find out what you really want to get out of it. Ask yourself, "Why do I *want* to do this? Why do I *need* this improvement?"

Write down your first reaction, then repeat that same question to yourself at least 2 more times, and allow yourself to dig deep and find the true answers.

The answers you find are now the beginning of your *Circulation Domination!* journey. They are your goals.

Let's call this your *Circulation Domination!* journal.

The *Circulation Domination!* Journal

There are 4 easy steps to keeping a *Circulation Domination!* journal. Do them and you will be intrigued by what you find.

Most of us go about our days rather mechanically—we get up, get dressed, eat breakfast (maybe), get the kids off to school, get ourselves off to work, come home, eat, get the kids to bed, watch TV, go to sleep. We get up and do it again, and again, and again ... But there are many things, sometimes tiny things, that we do or don't do that have big effects on our overall health and well-being.

Keeping a journal will help you uncover these unconscious items and take little steps that will result in big changes. In the final pages of *Circulation Domination!*, we're going to get you started on your journey by providing the outline for your journal.

Use what you have learned, make plans and take strides each day, and track your progress. With just a little effort, you will improve circulation, helping you look and feel better than ever.

Circulation Domination! Journal - Step 1

1. Start with an entry outlining what the journal is about, what your goals are, and how you plan to achieve them. Use the results of your soul-searching exercise as the basis for this first journal entry.

For example, if you're like me when I first started, your first journal entry may be similar to this:

> *"I'm tired of being tired. I'm tired of being lazy. I'm afraid that I will grow and look old before my time because I don't take care of myself like I should. I know there are things that I can do to help, so I am going to get up and DO THEM!*

> *"I've always felt like there was a fit, healthy, vibrant person inside of me, but I make too many excuses for not doing what it takes to let her shine. It's time to let her shine. I know I can do this.*

> *"I will start with small steps and make a promise to myself and my family to continue taking more and more steps. I will be healthy. I will feel better. I will look better. I can't wait to get started!"*

Once you have outlined the reasons for your goals, your goals themselves, and how you plan to achieve them, you are ready to start your journey.

Circulation Domination! Journal

In Step 1 of your *Circulation Domination!* journal, list why you are doing this and what you hope to accomplish.

I'm on a quest for Circulation Domination! because ...

_____
_____
_____
_____
_____
_____
_____
_____
_____

My goals are ...

_____
_____
_____
_____
_____

I plan to achieve them by doing/changing/starting ...

_____
_____
_____
_____
_____
_____

Circulation Domination! Journal - Step 2

2. Each day upon rising, note how you feel both mentally and physically. Note the day of the week and the date, and what you're setting off to do that day. Note the weather, too. (There are definite correlations between the weather and the way one feels!) Decide what *Circulation Domination!* goals you hope to achieve that day.

Try grouping your daily goals into three categories:

- **Hydration**
- **Nutrition**
- **Physical Activity**

Also add any changes you plan on implementing. Start small. If your goals are too high, you may not reach them, which could lead to disappointment—a surefire recipe for failure. Challenge yourself, but be realistic.

Throughout the day try to make several entries in your journal. Include what you eat. No need to count calories or be judgmental, just make a note of what you eat. Write down your activities, from the mundane to the physically challenging: showering, walking, taking the stairs instead of the elevator, scrubbing the bathroom, whatever you do. Note the mental ups and downs of the day, and what triggered them. Work, the kids, money, the news: there are many stress factors and triggers that we encounter during the day. Noting when they happen and your reaction to them can help you either avoid them in the future or deal with them in a way that takes less of a toll on your health.

End the day—just before you retire for the night—with a note about how you're feeling and how the day went. Always end on a positive note! Even if you didn't accomplish all that you set out to, you surely accomplished something. Allow yourself some positive feedback for what you did well. Set some preliminary goals for the following day.

Using Visuals in Your Journal Entries

When taking steps to make changes in your lifestyle, it is helpful to note what triggers certain behavior. Many people claim to overeat due to stresses in their lives, or things that happen throughout the day that trigger their emotional need to eat.

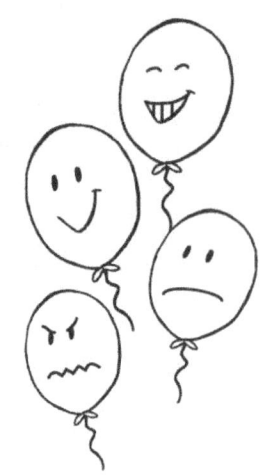

Making journal entries each day is a great way to uncover these triggers. Make a visual representation of how you feel each day in the morning and at night with little "emoticons"—simple icons that represent your emotions. Note how you feel with a happy face, a straight face, a sad face, or a mad face. Or, use whatever visual representations suit you best. It may seem silly at first, but it's actually quite interesting to look back over the week and see how you were feeling each morning and each night. Your emotional patterns may surprise you. They may also help explain your physical patterns.

Circulation Domination! Journal

In Step 2 of your *Circulation Domination!* Journal, begin making your daily journal entries.

Day 1

Date: _____ Day of the Week: _____

Today's Weather: _____

How I'm Feeling Today

_____

_____

_____

Today's Goals (Hydration, Nutrition, Activity)

_____

_____

_____

_____

Today's Notes & Accomplishments

_____

_____

_____

_____

_____

Summary & Notes for Tomorrow

_____

_____

_____

_____

_____

_____

Day 2

Date: _____ Day of the Week: _____

Today's Weather: _____

How I'm Feeling Today

☺ ☺ ☹ 😠

_____

_____

_____

Today's Goals (Hydration, Nutrition, Activity)

_____

_____

_____

_____

Today's Notes & Accomplishments

_____

_____

_____

_____

_____

_____

Summary & Notes for Tomorrow

_____

_____

_____

_____

_____

_____

_____

_____

Day 3

Date: _____ Day of the Week: _____

Today's Weather: _____

How I'm Feeling Today

_____

_____

_____

Today's Goals (Hydration, Nutrition, Activity)

_____

_____

_____

_____

Today's Notes & Accomplishments

_____

_____

_____

_____

Summary & Notes for Tomorrow

_____

_____

_____

_____

_____

_____

_____

Day 4

Date: _____ Day of the Week: _____

Today's Weather: _____

How I'm Feeling Today

_____

_____

_____

Today's Goals (Hydration, Nutrition, Activity)

_____

_____

_____

_____

Today's Notes & Accomplishments

_____

_____

_____

_____

_____

Summary & Notes for Tomorrow

_____

_____

_____

_____

_____

_____

_____

Day 5

Date: _____ Day of the Week: _____

Today's Weather: _____

How I'm Feeling Today   😛 😊 🙁 😠

_____

_____

_____

Today's Goals (Hydration, Nutrition, Activity)

_____

_____

_____

_____

_____

Today's Notes & Accomplishments

_____

_____

_____

_____

_____

_____

Summary & Notes for Tomorrow

_____

_____

_____

_____

_____

_____

_____

_____

Day 6

Date: _____ Day of the Week: _____

Today's Weather: _____

How I'm Feeling Today

_____

_____

_____

Today's Goals (Hydration, Nutrition, Activity)

_____

_____

_____

_____

Today's Notes & Accomplishments

_____

_____

_____

_____

_____

Summary & Notes for Tomorrow

_____

_____

_____

_____

_____

_____

_____

Day 7

Date: _____ Day of the Week: _____

Today's Weather: _____

How I'm Feeling Today   😃 😊 🙁 😠

_____

_____

_____

Today's Goals (Hydration, Nutrition, Activity)

_____

_____

_____

_____

Today's Notes & Accomplishments

_____

_____

_____

_____

_____

Summary & Notes for Tomorrow

_____

_____

_____

_____

_____

_____

_____

Circulation Domination! Journal - Step 3

3. At week's end, flip back through your entries for the week. Look at your visuals. Look at the ups and downs of your week. Look at the stress triggers that played a role in your mood.

End the week with a synopsis entry about how the week went, and the things you think may be hurting or helping your overall well-being. Also at the end of the week, tally your emoticons. Your goal, of course, should be to have many more happy ones than sad or mad ones. If it's weighted in the wrong direction, take a look back at the triggers that may have been at play. Your goals for the following week should include ideas for positively dealing with the triggers that have you down.

Keep your emoticon log for at least 4 weeks and note your physical and mental progress. If you are making positive changes to your lifestyle, setting goals and tracking your progress, you should be seeing positive results right away. If week after week your journal shows that you are more sad than happy, it may be time to speak with your doctor or a professional for help.

Circulation Domination! Journal

In Step 3 of your *Circulation Domination!* Journal, take a look back at the week's goals and accomplishments, and make a plan for next week.

My Weekly Summary

This week's ups, downs and emotional triggers, and list your accomplishments.

_____

_____

_____

_____

_____

_____

_____

_____

_____

Tally Your Emoticons!

How many happy, sad, mad or indifferent days did you have this week?

_____

_____

_____

My Goals for Next week

_____

_____

_____

_____

_____

_____

_____

_____

Circulation Domination! Journal – Step 4

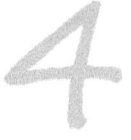 Continue making journal entries until you reach your personal goals. Consider it the handbook for your life, giving you insights, suggestions, and encouragement to make real, lifelong changes.

Even after you reach your goals, keep journaling whenever you feel the need. Use it to get back on track if you slip, or just as a way of staying in control.

Congratulations!

You are now on your way to *Circulation Domination!* I wish you the best and would love to hear about your progress!

Connect with me through the *Circulation Domination!* blog at www.CirculationDomination.com or via social media at www.facebook.com/circulationbook, and www.twitter.com/circulationbook.

ABOUT THE AUTHOR

Maryland native Kris McCurry is a forty-five-year-old wife and mom living just outside of Baltimore. A marketing professional turned author, Kris is a health and fitness fanatic, always seeking new information on staying fit.

During the winter of 2009, Kris had a serious case of the "winter blues." Run-down, unmotivated, and feeling sad, she was starting to feel old. After her doctor said that one of the best ways to beat the winter blues was to increase physical activity, she did, and in the process shook the blues, lost weight, and began to feel better than she had in years.

Kris's curiosity was piqued. How could increasing physical activity have such a profound effect not only on the body, but also the mind? Kris did some research on her overall improvement, and all signs pointed to circulation. The more research she did, the more she realized how critical circulatory health is, and how many ailments can be alleviated by taking care of it. And so the concept for the book was born.

"I hope that you found the book intriguing and are inspired to take the steps necessary to achieve your own Circulation Domination!"

—*Kris McCurry*

www.ingramcontent.com/pod-product-compliance
Lightning Source LLC
Chambersburg PA
CBHW070159290526
45789CB00002B/831